MANAGING YOUR CHILD'S CROHN'S DISEASE OR ULCERATIVE COLITIS

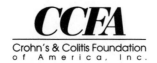

Crohn's & Colitis Foundation
of America, Inc.

Managing Your Child's Crohn's Disease or Ulcerative Colitis

BY
Keith J. Benkov, M.D.
AND
Harland S. Winter, M.D.

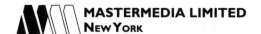

MASTERMEDIA LIMITED
New York

ISBN: 1-57101-023-0

Designed by Michael Woyton
Manufactured in the United States of America
10 9 8 7 6 5 4 3 2 1

I would like to thank a special group of people, sometimes referred to as patients, who have been crucial in teaching me, and without whom this book would not have been possible. I would also like to thank a second special group of people, always important to everything I do: my family. My wife, Judy, and my children, Carly and Jordan, provide me with the balance and perspective I need to do the work I love. — *KJB*

I would like to thank my cousin, Dr. Leon Goldman, who had Crohn's disease and encouraged me to enter the profession he loved; my children — Rachel, Michael, and Benjamin — for teaching me the importance of laughter, relaxation, and sports, especially soccer; and my wife, Susan, for her thoughtfulness, encouragement, love, and, most importantly, for sharing the passion she has for the happiness of all children. — *HSW*

ACKNOWLEDGMENTS

Medical knowledge is derived not only from written literature, but from listening closely to the experiences of patients and colleagues. For a long time now many medical practitioners have shared their insights about inflammatory bowel disease so that children and families and their doctors can learn about and improve its treatment. As authors and doctors, we have certainly benefited from this practice.

Particularly significant contributions to this book were made by members of the Pediatric Affairs Committee of the Crohn's & Colitis Foundation of America, Inc. (CCFA). Our special gratitude is extended to Susan S. Baker, M.D., Ph.D., Athos Bousvaros, M.D., Kathleen A. Calenda, M.D., Richard B. Colletti, M.D., Fred Daum, M.D., Anne M. Davis, R.D., Stephen Dolgin, M.D., Douglas A. Drossman, M.D., George D. Ferry, M.D., Mary-Joan Gerson, Ph.D., Richard J. Grand, M.D., Melvin B. Heyman, M.D., Stuart S. Kaufman, M.D., Barbara S. Kirschner, M.D., William J. Klish, M.D., Neal S. LeLeiko, M.D., Ph.D., Craig Lillehei, M.D., Susan N. Peck, R.N, David A. Piccoli, M.D., Nancy Rayhorn, R.N., C.G.R.N., Lynnae Schwartz, M.D., Robert C. Shamberger, M.D., Mitchell D. Shub, M.D., Claire Thibeault, R.N., John N. Udall, Jr., M.D., Ph.D., Jon A. VanDerhoof, M.D., Barry K. Wershil, M.D., and Rose J. Young, R.N., M.S. In addition, Robert A. Brine, National President of CCFA, National Director of CCFA, Barbara T. Boyle, and actress and CCFA spokesperson Mary Ann Mobley, are also owed a debt of thanks for their contributions. Jim Romano did his best to keep us on schedule, providing both editorial commentary and organizational support. Renardo Barden edited this book.

We would like to thank our patients and their friends and relatives for enlivening our efforts by sharing some of their struggles. We have, in the interest of ensuring personal privacy, withheld their names. Yet this book would be duller and darker without their unique contributions. Finally, we would like to thank all our patients and their families. We have been their doctors. They have been our teachers.

CONTENTS

PREFACE

As a volunteer with the Crohn's & Colitis Foundation of America, Inc. (CCFA), some of my most difficult moments have occurred as a result of hearing about the pain and distress experienced by children and young adults with Crohn's disease or ulcerative colitis. Unfortunately, since these diseases tend to befall the young, such moments have been all too common.

Guilt and anger, hope and determination, the desire to understand these diseases and diminish their pain and impact: these are common responses and emotions all too familiar to those whose children are ill. They are familiar to me as well. I am the father of a daughter with Crohn's disease.

For these and other reasons, I am proud that CCFA brings hope and knowledge to thousands of inflammatory bowel disease patients and their families. CCFA's quest for a cure and its educational resources brighten the lives of many families, including my own.

Managing Your Child's Crohn's Disease or Ulcerative Colitis is the first complete pediatric resource for parents and families. In focusing on the manifestations and control of these diseases in children and adolescents, the authors of this book have organized a wealth of clear and instructive information. Certain to prove helpful to both parents and their children, it is, by far, the best educational aid of its kind I have ever seen.

Some of the most respected gastroenterologists and authorities in the field today have contributed to its success. I am obliged to them for sharing their expertise so completely. No doubt, others will be equally pleased.

Like many of the best and most useful health publications, this book contains invaluable comfort, advice, and information generally unavailable elsewhere. While it takes more than written material to eradicate suffering or cure disease, I hope this book will provide readers with a valuable resource until scientists and researchers announce a cure for these diseases. For that day to come, of course, we need your help. In whatever way you can, please join CCFA in its mission to consign these illnesses to the medical history books.

ROBERT A. BRINE
NATIONAL PRESIDENT, CCFA

FOREWORD

To the public I am known as an actress, a former Miss America, and a documentary film maker. In my family, I am a daughter, a sister, a wife, and a mother. But to you, dear friends, I am a fellow patient — someone who was diagnosed with Crohn's disease in her twenties. It is as someone who has traveled a long, often uncertain road with inflammatory bowel disease (IBD) that I write to you.

My message to every child, teenager, and parent is a simple one. Never give up your dreams! Each of us is far more than just a patient. We are unique individuals who have so much to give to this world. Arm yourself with knowledge, learn to listen to and respect your body, and your dreams can be fulfilled.

When I was first diagnosed, a physician told me to give up acting. He said the stress would aggravate my Crohn's. I refused to listen to him and have enjoyed a wonderful career and a fabulous life. I worked with Elvis Presley in two films, received the Golden Globe award in 1965, and enjoyed several years as a member of "Circus of the Stars." I was a regular on "Diff'rent Strokes" and "Falcon Crest," and have appeared as a special guest on more than 100 TV shows. I also have traveled the world.

Back in the 1960s, I spent two memorable years living in Kenya while my husband, Gary Collins, starred in "Born Free." For many years I visited third world countries on behalf of World Vision. After the fall of Pol Pot's communist regime, I was a member of the first American TV film crew to enter Cambodia. And all this time I had Crohn's disease!

Please don't think that I'm special. Many, many other people with Crohn's disease or ulcerative colitis have achieved their dreams, too. Some are successful actors. Others are professional athletes. I've met a respected physician and researcher, a jet fighter pilot, a farmer, a forest ranger, and countless business people who have IBD.

Do we have our ups and downs? Of course we do! Do we sometimes become angry and depressed? You better believe it! But all of us have learned three things that have served us well. First, we have learned as much as we possibly can about IBD. We have become partners with our doctors in our treatments. Second, we have never tried to hide our illnesses. We talk to fellow sufferers and to anyone who cares to listen! Invariably, our lives are enriched by all the wonderful people we meet. And finally, we have never given up. We keep believing in ourselves, and in our dreams. Though our dreams may change, or our lives may take us in directions we never anticipated, we look back and find we have lived lives full of special memories of family, friends, and careers.

Remember us on those days that seem so bleak. The bad days will pass. And when they do, you will still have your dreams to fulfill.

MARY ANN MOBLEY

INTRODUCTION

This book is intended to help the 300,000 children with Crohn's disease and ulcerative colitis by informing them and their parents about inflammatory bowel disease. It has been written in the belief that knowledge empowers families and patients with the ability to make informed medical decisions about matters which affect their lives.

Since Crohn's disease and ulcerative colitis often present many different symptoms, these diseases are easily confused with other closely related gastrointestinal ailments, complaints, and conditions.

The body is not transparent and does not always produce clear, uniform symptoms when disease is present. In addition, the extent of a child's language development, the child's age, fears, and anxieties are often such that doctors must proceed toward a diagnosis without the benefit of reliable and consistent first-hand reports of symptoms. For these and other reasons, diagnosing and treating inflammatory bowel disease in children can be among the most difficult aspects of medicine.

The intestine absorbs food which our bodies store as fat, protein, and carbohydrates to be used at a later date for energy or growth. Most people think of this as its major role. Fewer realize that the gastrointestinal or GI tract is also the largest immune organ in the body. The immune system of the gastrointestinal tract protects us from viral, bacterial, and parasitic infections.

Unfortunately, it also happens that in addition to fighting infections, the immune system can react against the tissues of the intestine, causing injury. When a food causes this to happen, the condition is, at times, described as a 'food intolerance' or 'food allergy.' Usually, these sorts of intestinal injuries are resolved once the offending food is removed from the diet. However, the immune system in the GI tract sometimes becomes activated and associated with injury and inflammation unrelated to a specific food or infection for reasons that are not clear. Gastrointestinal symptoms that do not respond to dietary changes, can be associated with the condition called inflammatory bowel disease (IBD).

The causes of this ongoing inflammation of the gastrointestinal tract are unknown. Unfortunately, symptoms and medications often impact a child's growth and ability to participate in school activities. Along with experiencing physical pain and discomfort, some children with inflammatory bowel disease may also suffer from a diminished sense of security and well being.

Whenever a child complains of an illness, particularly one that may prove to be inflammatory bowel disease, children, families and doctors sometimes find themselves faced with the need to make decisions about testing and therapy. If the complaints are vague or symptoms relatively mild, decisions about the timing of various medical tests used to diagnose IBD can become complex. Because the child may have a transitory infection, the decision to proceed with diagnostic tests, however, is best made after obtaining a thorough history and making a careful examination of the child. The need for these time-consuming and sometimes painful medical tests should be discussed with patients and their parents as they become necessary.

As a group, children often have difficulty describing their symptoms clearly. Consequently, for parents and doctors, an assessment of changes in a child's play, behavior, or appetite may be more reliable indicators of problems than a description of symptoms. Listening carefully to observations made by family members, teachers, or friends, can be helpful to a doctor when attempting to reach a diagnosis or evaluating the success of a medical therapy already being provided to a sick child. Some children, of course, are better at describing symptoms and responses than others. In any case, doctors meeting with the child for the first time will want to know what sort of pain is being experienced and where it seems to be coming from. They will want to know if eating exacerbates or diminishes the pain, or if bowel pain is reduced by defecation. Does the child experience rectal cramping or "phantom" urges to pass stool? Since many gastrointestinal problems in children are caused by viruses, bacterial infections, and certain foods, doctors will want to know when the pain first started, and if anyone else in the family has been or is sick. If the child has been eating less, has there been a loss of weight? Are there signs of slowed physical growth? Is school performance or participation in social activities decreasing? Is there a family history of intestinal problems in general, or inflammatory bowel diseases in particular? These inquiries can be of considerable importance.

Following a diagnosis of IBD, many families are simply relieved that a diagnosis has been made. Such a response may be followed by a sense of frustration that the diagnosis was not made earlier and that such a disease has struck a previously healthy child. Children and parents should take the time to learn all they can about IBD. In so doing, they can become active participants in decisions to be made about medical care. To become more actively involved in medical decisions, families and patients must acquire a reasonable understanding of the disease process. Unfortunately, they must begin this process while learning to deal with the emotional impact of living with a chronic illness, one for which there is neither a single clearly identifiable cause nor a reliable cure. This cannot be an easy task. For families with IBD, there may be times of discouragement and setbacks. With the empowerment that comes from a knowledge of the disease, however, episodes of despair can be followed by periods of health, happiness, and renewed hope.

Fortunately, families and patients are not alone. The Crohn's & Colitis Foundation of America, Inc. (CCFA), provides IBD families with valuable educational materials, as well as access to seminars and support groups. Of course, no organization or book can provide the medical treatment and the steady, regular help needed by a child or adolescent with inflammatory bowel disease. Although we hope this book will prove to be a beneficial resource, we also wish to emphasize that treatment by a qualified doctor and close medical supervision are of prime importance.

What is Crohn's disease and how does it differ from ulcerative colitis? What does a patient's history have to do with the possibility he or she may have contracted inflammatory bowel disease? What can a doctor learn from a physical examination? What is the role played by laboratory and diagnostic tests? What other diseases and intestinal infections mimic IBD and create uncertainty about a patient's condition? How does a doctor go about determining whether a patient has Crohn's or ulcerative colitis? And, given the fact that the causes and cures of these diseases are unknown, how can physicians go about helping patients and families lead happy, healthy, and productive lives?

This book will address these questions. In the process, it will emphasize how inflammatory bowel disease varies from child to child. It will provide discussions that touch on the difficulties of interpreting medical findings. While reading this book, please remember that IBD does not lend itself to generalized descriptions. Although doctors may employ many different examination techniques in an effort to learn more about a child's disease, the course of ulcerative colitis and Crohn's disease are difficult to predict. Drugs that treat IBD can be effective for a period of time, and then mysteriously lose their capacity to bring relief. Perhaps almost as often, medications that bring no initial symptomatic relief, sometimes mysteriously begin to reduce symptoms. By understanding all they can about these diseases, families and children can actively participate with health care providers in finding and following a form of therapy that controls symptoms and restores quality of life.

PART I

DIAGNOSING INFLAMMATORY BOWEL DISEASE

CHAPTER I

INFLAMMATORY BOWEL DISEASE: AN OVERVIEW

ABOUT CROHN'S DISEASE AND ULCERATIVE COLITIS

Crohn's disease and ulcerative colitis are two separate but closely related diseases characterized by inflammation of the bowel or intestine. Neither disease is infectious or transmissible to other individuals; neither is entirely confined to the bowel; both tend to strike younger people. In addition to many gastrointestinal symptoms, both these diseases often result in extraintestinal symptoms, surprising disturbances outside the GI tract. Finally, both diseases generate gastrointestinal symptoms greatly resembling those of viral or bacterial infections, allergies, and other conditions. Given these similarities, as well as similarities of medical treatment, ulcerative colitis and Crohn's disease are often grouped together as inflammatory bowel disease (IBD).

Crohn's disease is currently without a cure, while ulcerative colitis is curable only through major surgery. Despite continuing research, the cause or causes of Crohn's disease and ulcerative colitis tend to be incompletely understood by the medical community. Nevertheless, the search for cures for these diseases goes on daily, even as new and increasingly successful methods of treatment are developed.

Physicians, along with the general public, may be puzzled or misinformed about these diseases. Crohn's disease and ulcerative colitis are real diseases, not syndromes. They are not the same as "spastic colitis," better known as irritable bowel syndrome, a condition experienced at times by as many as 25% of adult Americans. Crohn's disease and ulcerative colitis are not vague neurotic complaints or ailments brought on by poor eating habits. Neither are they induced by stress or diet or caused by psychological factors.

WHAT IS CROHN'S DISEASE?

Crohn's disease is an inflammatory illness involving any segment of the gastrointestinal tract from the mouth to the anus. An intestine inflamed by Crohn's disease may bleed, become narrowed, or blocked. The affected regions of the GI tract may be extensive or may be limited to an area of less than an inch. Despite medical treatment, a Crohn's-related inflammation may persist for a long period of time. Sometimes an area of inflammation heals spontaneously, without medical treatment. More often than not, however, inflammation is a recurrent problem. The symptoms of Crohn's disease that a child might experience vary from individual to individual and may change over time. Among these symptoms are cramping, abdominal pain, and diarrhea, loss of appetite and weight, a failure to grow as might be expected, persistent undernutrition, fatigue, fever, and vomiting. Stools may be hard and produce constipation, but often they are loose and may include blood. Some bloody stools can be seen with the naked eye, but not all blood in the stool is immediately visible. Special testing may be required to detect the presence of blood in fecal matter.

While the disease itself is old, its name is comparatively recent. In 1932, Burrill Crohn, M.D., Leon Ginzburg, M.D., and Gordon Oppenheimer, M.D., three doctors at Mount Sinai Hospital in New York, published a paper establishing Crohn's disease as a disease distinct from intestinal tuberculosis. For a time thereafter, Crohn's disease was classified according to the location of the inflammation. If areas of the small intestine were affected, the term regional enteritis was used. Inflammation of the end of the ileum was called ileitis or Eisenhower's disease (after the late President Eisenhower, who had Crohn's disease). Involvement of the colon or large intestine was referred to as granulomatous colitis in order to distinguish it from ulcerative colitis. The term Crohn's disease is now commonly used, irrespective of its location. However, since a child with Crohn's disease of the small intestine will experience different symptoms from those with inflammation of the colon or large intestine, the precise location of the disease is a matter of medical importance. Clinicians continue to describe Crohn's according to its location in the bowel.

WHAT IS ULCERATIVE COLITIS?

Ulcerative colitis is a chronic inflammation confined to the innermost lining of the large intestine. Most children with ulcerative colitis have bloody stools and abdominal pain. Although doctors have long sought an infectious cause for ulcerative colitis, no known bacterium, virus, parasite, or fungus has been found to cause this disease. However, children with a viral or bacterial infection may experience symptoms resembling various infections and conditions. Because ulcerative colitis is always confined to the large intestine, an x-ray revealing inflammation of the small intestine may strongly suggest the presence of Crohn's disease. However, Crohn's disease can also affect the inner lining of the large intestine. When Crohn's disease occurs in the large intestine, doctors may be unable, for a while, to determine whether a child has Crohn's disease or ulcerative colitis. Over time, Crohn's disease and ulcerative colitis tend to acquire distinct characteristics. If a child has an inflammatory bowel disease, eventually doctors will almost certainly be able to diagnose either Crohn's disease or ulcerative colitis. Fortunately for the child, medical treatment can often be instituted before a definitive diagnosis has been entered.

STEPS TOWARD A DIAGNOSIS OF INFLAMMATORY BOWEL DISEASE

Confronted with a child experiencing gastrointestinal symptoms of uncertain origin, a doctor might need to conduct a six-phase, multi-faceted investigation. In attempting to reach a diagnosis, it may be necessary for the doctor to:

1. Suspect IBD based on the results of a patient's history and a physical exam.
2. Perform a series of laboratory blood tests and stool cultures, thereby attempting to eliminate the possibility a child is suffering from other diseases.
3. Conduct more complex, invasive examinations and tests as needed in order to find out which areas or parts of the intestine are involved .
4. Analyze all the information gathered and determine whether the child has Crohn's disease or ulcerative colitis.
5. Discover if the child is also experiencing other conditions, diseases, or IBD-related extraintestinal symptoms that might affect a course of treatment.
6. Arrive at and provide the treatment best suited to the child's present condition.

WHO DEVELOPS INFLAMMATORY BOWEL DISEASE?

The Crohn's & Colitis Foundation of America (CCFA) estimates that about 2,000,000 Americans suffer from inflammatory bowel disease. Of these, perhaps 300,000 are in the pediatric age groups. The vast majority of newly diagnosed children with IBD are between 10 and 20 years of age. Interestingly, fewer than 5% of newly diagnosed IBD cases are discovered in children under 5. This makes Crohn's disease and ulcerative colitis common among the young, but rare among the very young. Nevertheless, these numbers do not tell all there is to know about who may develop inflammatory bowel disease. Virtually anyone, male or female, young or old, can develop IBD at any time.

A TENDENCY TO INHERIT INFLAMMATORY BOWEL DISEASE

Inflammatory bowel disease is not inherited in the way some diseases and many physical characteristics and personal traits are, but a family history of Crohn's disease or ulcerative colitis plays a role in the development of IBD. Studies have shown, for example, that Crohn's disease or ulcerative colitis can be expected to develop in approximately 10% of those with a first-degree relative (mother, father, offspring, or sibling) who has one of these diseases. If a parent has inflammatory bowel disease, there is a small (1 to 3%) chance that a child will also develop it. If both parents have IBD, the risk is somewhat higher. Identical twins are the most susceptible. If one twin has Crohn's, the other twin has about a 60% chance of also developing the disease. However, twins share ulcerative colitis only about 6% of the time. This suggests that genetic factors may play a more important role in Crohn's disease than ulcerative colitis.

While family members face greater risks of acquiring inflammatory bowel disease than individuals from families in which there is no history of Crohn's disease or ulcerative colitis, the increased risks are comparatively slight, and the odds are good that another family member will not acquire IBD. Disease-free individuals in a family in which there is a history of inflammatory bowel disease should do all they can to avoid worrying. Admittedly, this is easier said than done. However, since these diseases are not contagious and it has never been shown that worrying or trying to take extra precautions can prevent the diseases from occurring, family members will want to avoid unavailing anxiety.

Environmental and other factors also seem to exert some influence on the development of Crohn's or ulcerative colitis. For instance, Americans of Jewish ancestry are known to have a rate of incidence of inflammatory bowel disease about three times higher than the national average. Surprisingly, though, the incidence of Crohn's disease and ulcerative colitis in Israel is lower than in America. Thus it would appear that Israeli Jews are less at risk than American Jews. While people of northern European and Mediterranean descent are at higher than average risk, the incidence of IBD among Asians and Africans is low. Yet whenever Asians or Africans emigrate and resettle in western societies, the incidence of IBD appears to increase. Although the reasons for these latter patterns are unknown, the suggestion would seem to be that diet and environment play at least a limited role in their development.

PROPOSED ASSOCIATIONS AND RISK FACTORS FOR IBD

I. **Genetic**
   Northern European
   Jewish ancestry
   Family history

II. **Exogenous/dietary factors (no conclusive proof)**
   Milk consumption
   Sugar consumption
   Smoking
   Oral contraceptive pill

III. **Infectious (no conclusive proof)**
   Clostridium difficile
   Atypical mycobacterium
   Enteric bacterial flora
   Measles virus

IV. **Immune**
   Altered intestinal permeability
   Associated autoimmune diseases

(adapted with permission from Bousvaros and Walker, Gastrointestinal and Liver Disease, in Stiehm ER, *Immunologic Disorders of Infants and Children,* 4th Edition.)

THE DISCREDITED PSYCHOLOGICAL FACTOR

Once it was widely believed that psychological factors produced IBD. Despite the fact that these views have been discredited by many studies, the idea that these illnesses have a psychological component continues to be discussed in psychiatric literature. Indications are that while psychological factors do not cause these diseases, psychological factors do seem to influence immune system responses in some people. It is also likely that psychological factors have an impact on an individual's ability to cope with preexisting disease and with exacerbated symptoms. The view that psychological factors may play a small but unknown role in either the development, timing, or severity of inflammatory bowel disease symptoms has been somewhat strengthened by data suggesting that flare-ups of IBD symptoms may be more frequent or become more troubling during times of personal stress. The exact relationship between the immune system, stress, and flare-ups of IBD, however, is far from clear. Certainly neither children nor older patients should ever be made to feel that their disease symptoms are caused or aggravated by anxiety or psychological problems.

CHAPTER 2

SYMPTOMS AND A FIRST VISIT TO THE GASTROENTEROLOGIST

The more a child and parents understand about inflammatory bowel disease symptoms, the better prepared they will be to assist the doctor in reaching a diagnosis and participating in treatment. For that reason, we are including here a brief discussion of the significant symptoms of IBD. The most relevant and common gastrointestinal symptoms of inflammatory bowel disease are diarrhea, abdominal pain (whether or not associated with the passing of stool), and rectal bleeding. Weight loss or delayed growth, accompanied by a lack of sexual maturation, may also be sources of concern. These may or may not be accompanied by nausea, vomiting, fevers, rashes, joint pains, and mouth sores.

DIARRHEA

Both Crohn's disease of the small bowel and ulcerative colitis involving the colon can cause loose, watery stool, termed diarrhea. Because the small intestine is the part of the bowel where food is digested and absorbed into the body, inflammation of the small intestine can result in malabsorption with an accompanying loss of nutrients into the stool. These malabsorbed nutrients tend to carry extra water with them, making stools loose and watery. The main function of the large intestine is the reabsorption or recycling of water into the body. Whenever the large intestine is inflamed, water is not absorbed. Bowel movements become loose, resulting in diarrhea.

The doctor will want to know when the diarrhea started, how many bowel movements the child has been having per day, and if stool is being passed at night. If cramps or mucus accompany the passing of stool, or if cramps occur after the child has passed stool, this, too, can be important. Insofar as possible, the doctor will want to know how the diarrhea has changed over time, as well as how the diarrhea seems to be related to other symptoms such as fever, abdominal pain, or swelling of the abdomen. If stool exams have been conducted in the past, the doctor should be informed of their results. If anyone else at home has diarrhea, or if there has been recent family travel, this, too, may be significant. Sometimes diarrhea is caused by contaminated food or drink. In locales where the purity of the water supply may be questionable, the doctor may want to know if the patient drinks bottled or tap water.

ABDOMINAL PAIN

Whether or not it is associated with inflammatory bowel disease, abdominal pain can be highly subjective. Severe pain to one person can be tolerable to another. Exactly how the pain feels has nothing to do with how brave or tough a person is, so it will not serve the interests of the doctor if the child and parents dispute the intensity or frequency of the pain. From a medical standpoint, it is how the pain feels to the patient that is important.

Abdominal pain, which can take many different forms, is an important symptom of inflammatory bowel disease. For this reason, a child will be asked to note the exact location of pain. Particular attention will be paid to any pain that tends to move to different areas of the abdomen or back. Since inflammation of the stomach or esophagus are occasionally associated with Crohn's disease, pain above the umbilicus, particularly when accompanied by nausea, weight loss, poor growth, or delayed physical development, is likely to raise medical concerns about the possibility of inflammatory bowel disease. However, abdominal pain above the umbilicus may also be a sign of a peptic ulcer, pancreatitis, or gall bladder disease.

If a child's symptoms are centered in the lower right quadrant of the abdomen, the patient could be experiencing either appendicitis or the onset of an acute attack of Crohn's disease. Because the symptoms of inflammatory bowel disease and appendicitis can be quite similar, doctors operating for suspected appendicitis occasionally discover that a child's appendix is perfectly normal while the small intestine is thickened and narrowed. Although a diagnosis of Crohn's disease may be suspected on the basis of such a discovery, doctors must also exclude the possibility that the problems are being caused by intestinal bacteria known to mimic both Crohn's and appendicitis. Unlike Crohn's disease, which occurs often in the lower right region of the abdomen and so is sometimes confused with appendicitis, ulcerative colitis tends to cause more left-sided pain, often in the rectal area, and often associated with passing blood. Ulcerative colitis is highly unlikely to be mistaken for appendicitis.

Because of the complexity and importance of abdominal pain in the investigation of inflammatory bowel disease, specific descriptions of symptoms may be valuable to the doctor. Knowledge of how long the pain lasts, if it is constant or comes and goes, or if it occurs in spasms, may provide important diagnostic clues. Additionally, the doctor will want to know if the pain coincides with particular activities such as meals, if it starts or ends at a predictable time of day, or if it seems related in any way to a menstrual cycle. That the child's pain might be associated with a type of food is particularly relevant. If exercise, food, or certain types of stress seem to exacerbate the discomfort, what, if anything, seems to relieve it? Is the abdominal pain associated with fever or diarrhea? By giving some thought in advance to these topics, children and parents may be able to hasten diagnosis and treatment.

RECTAL BLEEDING

The onset of rectal bleeding and its relationship to other symptoms, especially diarrhea, is highly important. How much blood is being lost from the intestine? Are there clots in the toilet? If the child is not toilet trained, what is the size of the blood stain in the diaper?

The color of the blood being lost may provide additional clues about the location of the problem. Bright red blood, for example, usually comes from the end of the colon; black, tarry blood often originates from the stomach or upper small intestine; dark red blood may be traceable to the beginning of the colon or the end of the small intestine. Is the blood mixed with the stool, as it would tend to be in colitis, or is the formed stool coated with blood, as it might be if the patient had a polyp, fissure, or proctitis? Since blood irritates the bowel, if the child is bleeding during the night, he or she may be required to get up in order to pass a bloody stool. Under ordinary circumstances, the intestine, like the rest of the body, is inclined to relax at night. Therefore bloody stools passed at night may signal a more serious inflammation.

SLOW GROWTH

There are many causes of slow growth other than inflammatory bowel disease. Constitutional growth delay, for example, is a medical description sometimes employed to describe those who experience puberty at a later age than others. However, when delayed growth occurs in conjunction with bowel symptoms, doctors should be alerted to the possibility of inflammatory bowel disease.

On a day-to-day basis, children experiencing slow growth may simply be considered picky eaters. Certainly some young people are more choosy at the table and carefully select the number of foods they enjoy. However, over a period of months or years, an insufficient intake of calories may result in a form of slow growth often associated with inflammatory bowel disease.

Slow growth is one of the most subtle symptoms of inflammatory bowel disease and, where children are concerned, one of the most important. Many young people with only the mildest gastrointestinal complaints may be slow to acquire height, weight, and sexual maturity. For example, a boy once the tallest in his peer group, may slip to the middle of the class during adolescence. A girl of average size and weight might be surpassed in height and weight by all her friends.

EXTRAINTESTINAL SYMPTOMS

Other more general or systemic symptoms can also be important in the diagnosis of inflammatory bowel disease. Many of these conditions, often referred to as extraintestinal symptoms, occur in other illnesses and are not necessarily exclusively associated with either the gastrointestinal tract or IBD. In addition to joint pains, extraintestinal symptoms of inflammatory bowel disease may include fever, malaise (not feeling well), fatigue, an inability to keep up in school, and poor appetite.

COMPARISON OF SIGNS AND SYMPTOMS OF IBD*

(taken directly from A Physician's Guide to
Pediatric Crohn's Disease and Ulcerative Colitis)

ULCERATIVE COLITIS		CROHN'S DISEASE	Children	Adults
Diarrhea	90%	Abdominal Pain	82%	85%
Bleeding	90%	Diarrhea	88%	62%
Weight Loss	50%	Growth Failure	60-90%	—
Pain	80%	Fever	77%	41%
Arthritis	5%	Vomiting	10-30%	—
Growth Failure	14%	Arthralgias	23%	—
Fever	40%	Skin Problems	0-10%	—
		Rectal Bleeding	22%	13%
		Anorexia	0-30%	—
		Perianal Disease	25%	—
		Weight Loss	80-90%	50%

* Signs and symptoms depend on the location of disease.
(Adapted from Motil KJ, Grand RJ, Ulcerative colitis and Crohn's disease in Children. In: Kirsner JB, Shorter RG, eds. *Inflammatory Bowel Disease.* 3rd ed. Philadelphia: Lea and Febiger, 1988: 227.)

JOINT PROBLEMS

Some children with inflammatory bowel disease have joint pains, while others rarely, if ever, experience swelling or pain in these areas. Sometimes joints in the back are painful, causing a child to experience lower back pain. Most of the time, however, pain is located in the larger joints such as the hips, knees, shoulders, ankles, and wrists. In an effort to find out if a child's movements are in any way painful or being restricted by joint problems, the doctor may call on the child to perform some simple exercises of the arms, legs, and back. Unlike joint pains associated with rheumatoid arthritis, those experienced in IBD rarely disfigure children. They can, however, limit a child's activity.

MILDER CASES

A child may have Crohn's disease or ulcerative colitis without complaining of any of the dramatic symptoms usually associated with inflammatory bowel disease. It has been estimated that up to 33% of children diagnosed with inflammatory bowel disease have experienced mild symptoms for several months or even years before finally being diagnosed with IBD. The most persuasive rationale for these delays in diagnosis is that many symptoms may seem too mild to characterize a chronic disease. Then, too, some symptoms suggest other causes, such as allergic reactions to foods or bacterial or viral infections. Mild inflammatory bowel disease manifestations can be similar to those of rheumatoid arthritis, growing pains, or even anorexia nervosa. They might also include periodic low-grade fevers of between 100 and 101 degrees Fahrenheit, vague cramps or pains, abdominal tenderness when touched, loose stools, nausea, or general fatigue. Although some weight loss may have occurred, more often than not, in a child with mild symptoms, there may be a failure simply to gain the weight or height predicted by growth charts and a slowness to develop signs of maturity. Other features of subacute presentation might include mouth ulcers, discomfort when passing stools, large skin tags around the anus, discharge from the rectum, skin rashes (particularly painful red bumps on the shins), or joint pain, with or without swelling. Even if a child doesn't complain of bloody stools, a rectal exam may show large skin tags (redundant folds of skin) around the anus.

THE INITIAL VISIT: A PHYSICAL EXAMINATION

A child's first visit to a specialist who treats children with gastrointestinal problems is likely to be a source of anxiety and concern to the entire family. Parents in particular will have many questions. What is

---

PRESENTING FEATURES OF **IBD** IN CHILDHOOD

Intestinal
Growth failure
Weight loss
Diarrhea
Abdominal pain
Abdominal mass (a fullness felt by the doctor on examination)
Rectal bleeding (passing blood with bowel movements)
Fissures (or cracking around the rectum)

Extraintestinal (Outside the Intestine)
Arthritis or arthralgia (pain when moving joints)
Skin rashes
Fever
Anorexia (loss of appetite)
Recurrent mouth ulcers (canker sores)
Anemia (pale, sallow appearance)
Pubertal delay

(Adapted with permission from Bousvaros and Walker, Gastrointestinal and Liver Disease, in Stiehm ER, *Immunologic Disorders of Infants and Children,* 4th Edition.)

FEATURES OF PUBERTAL DELAY

BOYS	**GIRLS**
Lack of pubic hair and beard	Breasts do not develop
Penis does not grow with maturation	Periods do not start

---

the problem? Is it serious? Will the child lead a normal life? How did the problem develop?

Parents seeking reassurance are likely to meet with a doctor who seems reluctant to speculate about a child's problems in advance of a medical investigation. After doing what can reasonably be done to reassure and address the concerns of both child and parents, the doctor may have a great many questions to ask. The doctor is likely to begin by seeking details about the origins and precise nature of the child's symptoms.

Although specific written notes about a patient's pains and discomforts would prove helpful, a doctor understands that most parents don't report to the doctor's office with carefully compiled lists of dates and symptoms. Even so, parents and children will want to be as prepared for the initial interview as possible. When did the child's symptoms start? How often do they occur? How long do they last? How have they changed over time?

PREPARATION FOR THE VISIT

Providing a child with information about an initial doctor's appointment is important. A parent would do well to call the doctor's office and inquire in order to provide the child with information about what to expect during this first encounter. Will the child have to get undressed? What about a rectal examination? Will blood tests be performed? It is also true, of course, that while advance preparation for the first appointment will help many children cope with the sometimes uncomfortable experience of being examined, parents will want to exercise their own judgment. Providing too much information may succeed only in making some children anxious and reluctant to see the doctor.

Some doctors have difficulty staying on time because of busy schedules. Be prepared for this possibility by asking the receptionist in advance if the doctor is usually on time. Since even the most punctual doctors fall behind on occasion, it is a good idea for parents to bring along a book or quiet game. By providing the child with subdued personal attention and modest entertainment at the doctor's office, a parent can soothe a child's fears and keep anxieties from escalating.

Whether bowel symptoms are dramatic or mild, the doctor will want to talk to the child and conduct a thorough physical examination. Inquiries are likely to include requests for information about a child's height, weight, and growth rate. Did the child's growth start to slow down before gastrointestinal symptoms became troublesome? Weight loss or a failure to gain weight or height can be a sign of eating too little. But a slowness to grow can also indicate nutritional losses resulting from malabsorption of food. Body build, muscularity, and fat stores will be taken into account as the doctor makes efforts to discover if a child has nutritional deficiencies.

Whenever possible, your child's height and weight records should be brought to the doctor's office. Information about the height and weight of brothers and sisters, as well as parents and grandparents, may also be of value. The doctor may feel a need to consult growth charts in order to compare your child's stature with that of other children the same age. During an initial exam, the doctor will probably make a record of the child's height and weight. In measuring height, doctors often use centimeters. To convert centimeters to inches, divide by 2.54. For example, a young person whose height is recorded as 150 centimeters is about 59 inches or 4′11″ tall. Some doctors use kilograms to record weight. To convert kilograms to pounds, multiply by 2.2. For example, a child tipping the scale at 50 kilograms will weigh 110 pounds.

FINDINGS OUTSIDE THE GI TRACT

The joints are likely to be examined for signs of arthritic swelling that sometimes accompanies IBD. Since certain skin problems, such as red, bumpy swellings on the legs, are associated with inflammatory bowel disease, their appearance may be significant. Additionally, young patients will be inspected for mouth sores and rashes, as well as a spoon-shaped deformity of the nails known as clubbing.

THE RECTAL EXAMINATION

If there is blood in the stool, a physician will want to inspect the anal opening in search of tears or fistulas. Fistulas are ulcerations in the intestinal wall. These ulcerations may connect with other parts of the intestine, or with adjoining organs, or drain to the skin. While inspecting the anus and rectum, the doctor will also be looking for the pus-draining lesions often associated with Crohn's disease. Skin tags, or redundant folds of skin around the anal region, are also often linked with Crohn's disease.

An examination of the rectum is often an embarrassing experience for children. Not knowing what to expect from such an exam can increase the child's anxiety. If there is rectal inflammation, the insertion of a doctor's gloved finger can be painful. In such a situation, the doctor may make use of a special lubrication intended to numb the anal area. Most of the time, however, the exam is not painful and a regular lubricant is all that is necessary.

The rectal examination is an important part of the physical exam. Although a private part of the body is involved, children should be helped to understand the value of the procedure. By feeling inside the rectum with a rubber glove, the doctor may learn important information about a child's condition. Children who are able to help the doctor by lying quietly and explaining what is felt in response to the doctor's touch may provide great assistance. By looking at the outside of the anus, a doctor can sometimes discover clues about disease activity in the colon, particularly if there are skin tags or small growths around the rectum. Sometimes these growths are mistaken for hemorrhoids. Hemorrhoids, which are blue in color because they are blood vessels, may shrink when pushed. Skin tags look like extra flaps of skin and do not shrink when pressed. After the exam, the doctor may test the stool for blood that may not be visible to the naked eye.

A discussion of treatments for these inflammatory bowel symptoms will be found in chapter 8.

CHAPTER 3

LABORATORY TESTS

If the patient history and an initial physical exam do not eliminate the possibility that your child has inflammatory bowel disease, the doctor will probably call for further tests. Although complex and invasive diagnostic procedures sometimes become necessary, the doctor is likely to begin with investigations of blood, stool, and urine samples. These samples, obtained from your child by the doctor or medical assistants, will be submitted to special laboratories for evaluation and analysis.

It is important to understand both the usefulness and limitations of these laboratory tests. Blood and stool samples are evaluated for evidence of inflammation, indications of possible disease activity, and clues about what may be occurring in your child's gastrointestinal tract. Yet no one blood test or combination of tests will positively confirm the presence of IBD or pinpoint, precisely, a site of inflammation. Ideally, results from these tests will enable a doctor to carefully focus a diagnostic investigation.

BLOOD TESTS

When warranted, blood specimens are usually taken at the doctor's office by inserting a small needle into a vein and then drawing a small amount of blood. Because children often fear needles and bleeding, they may be unduly anxious about blood tests. The best preparation for a child faced with blood tests will vary from child to child and so is best left as a matter of parental discretion. Too much discussion of blood tests may result in fear and a desire not to go to the doctor's office. On the other hand, glib assurances that there will be no blood tests may give rise to feelings of parental betrayal and distrust if the doctor then deems such a test necessary. Unless you have received advance assurances from the doctor that blood tests will be unnecessary, promises are unwise. Honesty is important, but in this matter, honesty may not

17

require a somber, detailed discussion of blood tests. In most instances, parents will do better to tell a child that they do not know if blood will be taken, but that they will discuss the matter with the doctor. In addition, children should be helped to understand that, at times, blood must be tested to enable the doctor to provide the most effective form of treatment.

A child should be reassured that there is no connection between painful bowel symptoms and undesirable behavior. Never exploit a child's fears or use the doctor as an agent of parental discipline or punishment by employing the threat of a blood test in order to elicit desirable behavior from your child. Such a threat is cruel. It also exploits the vulnerability of children already susceptible to thinking of illness as a form of punishment visited on children who fail to meet parental standards. Your child may well need your help in understanding that gastrointestinal illness is not a form of punishment visited on "bad" or disobedient children.

Although doctors may at times call for other blood tests, the most frequently used tests in screening for inflammatory bowel diseases are the complete blood count (CBC), the erythrocyte sedimentation rate (ESR), and the serum albumin.

Routine screening of laboratory tests may result in a decision to do further studies or discontinue testing. In a child who seems well and is growing normally, with normal routine labs and stool tests, inflammatory bowel disease is unlikely. A child with persistent diarrhea and abnormal lab findings and/or occult blood in the stool, will probably be studied further. Obviously, a child who is ill enough to be in the hospital will be studied more quickly, regardless of lab findings.

LABORATORY EVALUATION OF PATIENTS WITH POSSIBLE IBD

Stool guaiac lab test for hidden blood in stool
CBC with differential, reticulocyte count
Sedimentation rate (test for inflammation)
Albumin, total protein
Liver function tests
Tests for iron deficiency
Antigliadin, anti-reticulin Ab, anti-endomysial Ab (to exclude celiac disease)
PPD/Candida skin tests (to exclude tuberculosis)
Stool cultures (for bacteria to exclude infection)
Stool analysis (for intestinal parasites)

(excerpted and adapted with permission from Bousvaros and Walker, Gastrointestinal and Liver Disease, in Stiehm ER, *Immunologic Disorders of Infants and Children*, 4th Edition).

Many children with inflammatory bowel disease will show some degree of anemia, with a low red blood cell count, a low hemoglobin, and a low hematocrit. All these values reflect the same measure — the quantity of red blood cells available. Hemoglobin is the actual protein within the red blood cell that carries oxygen, while hematocrit indicates how many red cells can be packed into a given volume of whole blood. Also included in the CBC test is a white blood cell count (WBC). Since white blood cells constitute one of the body's defenses against infection, the WBC is frequently elevated when the immune system is active in inflammatory bowel disease. The last major determinant of the CBC is the platelet count. Platelets are small cells that help the body to clot blood where there is a cut, an ulcer, or an area of inflammation. The platelet count, too, can be elevated in children with inflammatory bowel disease.

Typically, the erythrocyte sedimentation rate (ESR) or the C-reactive protein (CRP) blood tests simply tell the physician if there is inflammation somewhere in the child's body. Unfortunately, the tests do not indicate which part of the body is inflamed. Therefore, a child with hepatitis or inflammation of the liver can have the same degree of elevation of ESR as a child with inflammatory bowel disease. Furthermore, some children with IBD and active inflammation will still have a normal ESR.

Specific nutrient deficiencies can also be identified with blood tests. Because of the importance of good nutrition to healing inflamed areas of the intestine, discovering and treating any specific nutritional deficiencies is important to a child's care. Children are growing, and growth requires vitamins, minerals, protein, and calories. Not only does a vitamin deficiency impair the healing process, but it can also result in slow growth. Iron is absorbed in the segment of the small intestine not usually affected by Crohn's disease. However, blood loss associated with diarrhea often results in an iron deficiency. Hence, the iron normally present in some commonly eaten foods may fail to compensate for blood losses in the stool. In such instances, the child will develop a low hematocrit or hemoglobin. Vitamin B-12 is absorbed in the final portion of the small bowel (terminal ileum). This area is commonly inflamed in Crohn's disease. Whenever it is, the normal absorption of Vitamin B-12 can be impaired, resulting in a deficiency of this vitamin. Such a deficiency can also cause a low hematocrit or hemoglobin.

An inflammation of the gastrointestinal tract can cause serum proteins to weep from the inflamed lining and be carried off in the stool. When serum proteins are measured in the blood, the common ones being albumin and total protein, these values can be low because of losses in the stool. Owing to inflammation, other proteins, such as alpha-1-antitrypsin, will also be lost in the gastrointestinal tract and can be measured in the stool as a test of protein loss.

LABORATORY DIAGNOSIS OF DIARRHEAL ILLNESSES RESEMBLING IBD

Lab exams can be useful in identifying other diseases with symptoms similar to those of inflammatory bowel disease. Celiac disease or gluten enteropathy is a disease characterized by diarrhea and poor growth caused by an intolerance to wheat, barley, or rye. At times, the symptoms of celiac disease are confused with Crohn's disease. Three blood tests can be used to suggest or identify gluten enteropathy in children. These tests are anti-gliadin antibody, anti-reticulin antibody, and anti-endomysial antibody. These tests can also be positive in some children with Crohn's disease.

Diarrheal diseases caused by parasites can be detected by testing other antibodies in the blood. Antibodies are proteins manufactured in the immune system in order to fight off a specific infection. Some patients can have detectable antibodies indicating the possible presence of certain organisms responsible for intestinal infections like *Entamoeba histolytica, Yersinia,* and *Salmonella.* However, these serologic tests are not as reliable, diagnostically speaking, as stool tests. This is so because serologic tests do not tell the doctor if an infection is actually current. Since an immunologic response tends to persist in the blood long after the actual infection has disappeared, blood tests may continue to show evidence of, for example, Salmonella, long after the actual infection has ceased to be a factor in the child's overall health. For that reason, identifying an organism in the stool provides the best documentation that a child has an active infection.

In some patients, lab tests are conducted to exclude the possibility of generalized or systemic diseases such as rheumatological disease or tuberculosis. A PPD (purified protein derivative) is a skin test given by injecting with a needle a small amount of fluid under the skin. A bubble is raised and the area stings for a few seconds. If the area is red 48 hours later, the patient might have been exposed to tuberculosis. Since medications used to treat inflammatory bowel disease can exacerbate tuberculosis, it is important to be certain a child does not have tuberculosis before providing any of the medications used in treating inflammatory bowel disease.

If a child has symptoms suggestive of IBD, and neither visible nor occult blood is detected in the stool, the problem may be an inability to tolerate lactose, the sugar derived from milk products. Symptoms of lactose intolerance consist of bloating, cramps, and diarrhea, all suggestive of the possible presence of IBD. When a patient is unable to digest lactose properly, bacteria normally present in the intestine will digest. When bacteria digest the lactose, the presence of hydrogen gas can be detected in exhaled breaths. The breath is collected over a period of about three hours (every thirty minutes) after the child has consumed a glass of lactose. When a significant rise in the breath hydrogen levels occurs, lactose intolerance is diagnosed.

STOOL EXAMS: FECAL BLOOD

The presence of blood in the stool is one of the major findings in IBD. Having detected blood in the stool and eliminated the possibility that the child is suffering from an intestinal infection or from a localized irritation like a fissure or hemorrhoid, a doctor is likely to look further for inflammatory bowel disease. Even if there is no visible blood in the stool, there may be occult blood (detectable only through chemical or microscopic tests). Laboratory investigations of collected stool can provide a great deal of important information of this sort. Because of this, some doctors who treat young IBD patients make a practice of having stools checked for occult blood periodically, perhaps once every six to twelve months. Not only are such exams useful in monitoring treatments provided to inflammatory bowel disease patients, they are also helpful in detecting relapses which occur from time to time.

STOOL EXAMS: MICROORGANISMS

Stool exams also provide information about organisms often responsible for some diseases that mimic inflammatory bowel disease. As has been noted, intestinal infections lasting from one to ten days are often either viral or bacterial and may cause cramps and bloody diarrhea. Bacterial infections sometimes mistaken for IBD include *Salmonella, Shigella, Yersinia, Campylobacter, Clostridium difficile,* and *Escherichia coli.* Stools should also be studied for ova and parasites such as *Giardia, cryptosporidia,* and *amoeba.* These infections can persist undiagnosed for a long time unless patients undergo the stool exams intended to detect them. Since, for the most part, such infections are transmitted through contaminated food, impure water, or by contact with infected pets or farm animals, the doctor will want to know if other family members are sick. In addition, it will be important for the doctor to know if the child has traveled recently, or been exposed to potentially contaminated food, including meals from fast-food restaurants.

Has the child been taking antibiotics? If so, the antibiotics may have destroyed good intestinal bacteria along with the bad and, in the process, stimulated the overgrowth of an intestinal organism known as *Clostridium difficile.* Unchecked, this organism produces a toxin that causes an inflammation of the lining of the colon very similar to that which is seen with IBD. Although *Clostridium* is likely to have been caused by antibiotic usage, problems arising in connection with the organism's overgrowth can be successfully treated with other antibiotics.

When a medical history, a physical examination, and laboratory tests suggest a child may have inflammatory bowel disease, the doctor is likely to indicate the need for further testing. If an initial examination and laboratory testing fail to eliminate IBD as a possible explanation for your child's symptoms, the doctor will also probably want to look more carefully with other diagnostic tests.

CHAPTER 4

DIAGNOSTIC TESTS

As we have seen, a doctor evaluating a child with possible IBD will ordinarily begin with a personal medical history, proceed to a straightforward physical examination, and follow up by calling for some of the laboratory tests described in chapter 3.

Having come this far, of course, it is possible that the doctor will have eliminated the possibility that a child has inflammatory bowel disease and will already have instituted treatment for another condition.

If, however, the medical findings remain inconclusive after lab test results have been evaluated, the odds are the doctor will probably not speculate about your child's condition until after performing one or more of the diagnostic procedures described below. While essentially straightforward, the invasive examinations discussed in this chapter require sedation, advance preparation, and are often unpleasant. Because they can be uncomfortable and costly and will not, in and of themselves, resolve the child's condition, the doctor will want parents and children to understand their importance.

At issue here is striking the right balance between the doctor's need for more information about a child's medical condition, and the child's understandable desire to avoid these examinations if at all possible. Because the endoscopic examinations and x-rays described below are invasive and involve some anxiety and discomfort to the child, the doctor will want to perform these exams in a sensitive manner. In order to do so, the doctor will have given some thought to which procedures is most likely to yield the diagnosis and treatment options being sought. A basic overview of the gastrointestinal tract and how digestion works is important to understanding the doctor's efforts to learn about the conditions in your child's body.

THE GASTROINTESTINAL TRACT

The task of the gastrointestinal tract is to turn complex food into the micronutrients, proteins, fats, carbohydrates, vitamins, and minerals needed for normal body function. The gastrointestinal tract consists of the mouth, esophagus, and stomach, together with the small and large intestines. Associated with the gastrointestinal tract are major organs, namely the liver, pancreas, and gallbladder, whose function is to assist digestion. The small intestine, like a loopy garden hose, is connected both to the stomach and the large intestine. In adults, the small intestine can be as long as 18 feet. For descriptive purposes, the segment closest to the stomach is called the duodenum, while the long middle section is known as the jejunum, and the lowermost part is identified as the ileum. The ileocecal valve is the sphincter connecting the small intestine with the colon (large intestine). The colon, about a yard in length, is shaped somewhat like an inverted letter 'U.' The ileocecal valve connects with the large intestine above the cecum, a pouchlike structure which forms the first portion of the large intestine and from which hangs the appendix. The cecum becomes the ascending colon, which then turns at a sharp angle to become the trans-verse colon. It curves again, downward at a sharp angle, to become the descending colon. The descending colon opens into an enlarged tube known as the sigmoid colon, which then continues to descend into the rectum. The anus is the opening from which stool emerges.

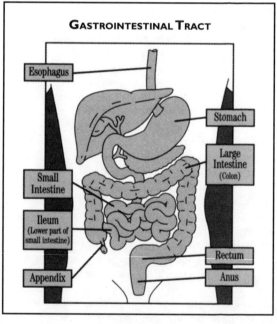

GASTROINTESTINAL TRACT

Esophagus

Stomach

Large Intestine (Colon)

Small Intestine

Ileum (Lower part of small intestine)

Appendix

Rectum

Anus

The tube forming the large and small intestines consists of four layers. The innermost layer is called the mucosa or the lining. Just below the mucosa is the submucosa. This is surrounded by the muscular layer known as the muscularis. The final layer, the serosa, forms a protective coating surrounding the other three layers. Together these layers make up the intestinal wall.

ABOUT DIGESTION

Digestion begins in the mouth assisted by salivation and chewing and continues as food is swallowed, passes through the esophagus, and into the stomach. From the stomach, food moves into the duodenum, the jejunum, and the ileum. As partially digested food is passed along by various muscles via a process known as peristalsis, many enzymes continue to break the food down into smaller particles. The task of the small intestine is to absorb these small particles and transport them via the bloodstream throughout the body. When the almost entirely digested mixture reaches the large intestine, water and salts are absorbed. The remaining waste is passed down through the large intestine and into the rectum where it is expelled from the anus in the form of stool.

The major work of digestion goes on in the small intestine, which lies just beyond the stomach. Digestive juices from the liver (bile) and the pancreas mix with food in the small intestine. The mixing is powered by the churning action of the intestinal muscle wall. Having been broken down into small molecules, digested food is absorbed through the small intestinal surface and distributed to the rest of the body by the blood stream. Watery food residue not digested in the small intestine passes into the large intestine, which reabsorbs much of the water previously added to food in the small intestine. This takes place through a kind of water conservation or recycling mechanism in the colon. Solid, undigested food residue is then passed from the large intestine as a bowel movement.

When the small intestine is inflamed, as it often is with Crohn's disease, the intestine becomes less able to fully digest and absorb the nutrients present in food. Depending on how extensively and how severely the small intestine is injured, such nutrients can, to varying degrees, escape into the large intestine. Though many children with IBD simply lack appetite and fail to eat enough, improperly digested food and malabsorbed nutrients are among the reasons children with inflammatory bowel disease become malnourished. Furthermore, incompletely digested foods traveling through the large intestine interfere with water conservation, even if the large intestine is not itself damaged. Thus, Crohn's disease affecting the small intestine may cause both diarrhea and malnutrition. If the large intestine is also inflamed, however, the resultant diarrhea is likely to be worse.

X-RAYS

X-rays play an important role in evaluating a child for possible inflammatory bowel disease. A simple snapshot of the abdomen known as a plain film or KUB (for kidneys, ureter, and bladder) may be helpful in determining whether or not these three important organs are involved in disease activity. X-rays can also demonstrate any unexpected dilation in the loops of the intestine and provide visual evidence as to whether or not fluids are moving properly. Kidney stones or gallstones are sometimes identified as well. X-rays of wrist bones and knees, known as bone age tests, can provide helpful information about growth patterns.

KUB

BONE AGE TESTS

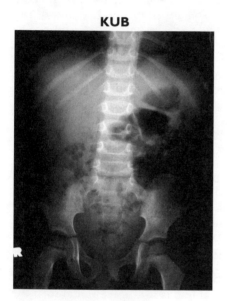 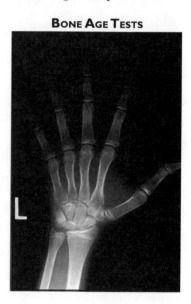

ABOUT BARIUM X-RAYS

While bones can be seen clearly on x-rays, the essentially hollow gastrointestinal tract is normally visible on plain x-ray only as a series of indistinct shadows where air outlines the inside of the bowel. Barium can resolve this problem. Once inside the GI tract, barium coats the inner lining of the bowel and shows distinctly white on film. Barium, a white, chalklike substance appears densely white on X-ray; hence doctors often speak of barium tests as "contrast studies." Barium x-ray films sometimes reveal a scarring or narrowing of the bowel. Fistulas, ulcers, and other lesions may also be detected.

Although it is uncomfortable for the child, the doctor may need to rely on barium (flushed into the rectum via an enema) in order to determine the exact location of inflammation within the bowel. The presence of barium in the bowel is rarely painful unless there is serious internal inflammation. Even so, young people may find barium unpleasant. Children scheduled for barium-assisted examinations will be limited to clear liquids for 24 to 48 hours prior to the exam, must go without food for several hours beforehand, and will be required to undergo a series of "clean-out" enemas or laxatives before undergoing the barium enema. These procedures are made necessary because any presence of stool or gas in the colon would obscure the view and perhaps prevent the doctor from making potentially important findings.

THE BARIUM ENEMA

A barium enema is an uncomfortable but ordinarily painless procedure. A catheter is inserted into the anus and fills the colon with the white solution. The injected liquid produces the sensation of needing to go to the bathroom. This, however, is not immediately necessary. In fact, if the exam is to be successful, the child will need to endure this impulse. From the distribution of the barium and the way it outlines the organs, a doctor will be able to detect any blockage, narrowing, or possible ulceration of the lining of the colon.

BARIUM ENEMA

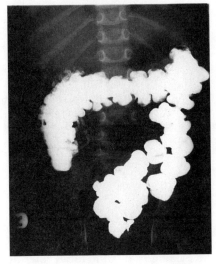

Although at times, a pediatrician will have ordered a barium enema prior to referring a patient to a specialist, these days barium-assisted examinations are less frequently called for by gastroenterologists. To a great extent, barium-assisted examinations have been replaced by advances in endoscopy, particularly endoscopic exams.

THE UPPER GI AND THE SMALL BOWEL SERIES

If a doctor suspects the presence of Crohn's disease in the uppermost sections of a child's gastrointestinal tract, an upper GI may be the doctor's examination of choice. This exam makes it possible for the doctor to view the barium-coated esophagus, stomach, and uppermost small intestine. The organs may be x-rayed one image at a time or viewed on a television-like monitor. In an upper GI, barium is given by mouth and its progress carefully viewed and followed all the way down. As the barium moves through the gastrointestinal tract, the doctor searches

SMALL BOWEL SERIES

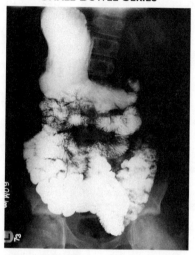

for signs of swelling, inflammation, fistulas, blockages, and other problems which may need medical treatment. As the barium flows down from the duodenum into the jejunum, ileum, and thence into the large intestine, additional images may be taken. Any narrowing or scarring will be carefully noted and evaluated. Because it is the most commonly affected area in Crohn's disease, the doctor will pay special attention to the final segment of the ileum. Detailed "spot" films may be taken to enable the doctor to carefully focus on discrete areas. In order to obtain a better view of this and other important areas, the doctor may need to push on the child's abdomen, thereby manipulating an area of the bowel obscuring the area of interest. Although this maneuver can be alarming and mildly uncomfortable to a child, it is a harmless procedure and has only a very temporary affect on the form or shape of a child's GI tract. Because narrowing and scarring and other intestinal obstructions can slow the movement of the barium, this procedure can take from two to four hours, or even longer.

ENDOSCOPIC EXAMS

In recent years the availability of endoscopy has greatly enhanced medical knowledge about the appearance of healthy and diseased conditions inside the bowel. In general, endoscopy ("endo" meaning inside, "scope," meaning look), refers to the passing of flexible tubes roughly the diameter of a large crayon, into the gastrointestinal tract. While the upper GI and small bowel series make it possible for doctors to see x-ray images of the barium-coated shapes of the digestive organs, endoscopic examinations enable doctors to examine the linings of these organs and to directly view surfaces that can be examined in almost no other way.

The endoscope is a multi-purpose instrument consisting of several internal channels. One fiberoptic channel provides light, while another transmits the images. Additional endoscopic channels make it possible for the endoscopist to cleanse the bowel with water or inflate the intestine with air (to more easily pass the instrument). Yet another channel allows for the insertion and passage of smaller instruments which enable a doctor to snip a piece of intestinal tissue for the purposes of a biopsy.

ABOUT ENDOSCOPIC BIOPSIES

Since there are no x-ray or blood tests that definitely establish a diagnosis of inflammatory bowel disease, tissue biopsies may be needed to exclude diseases that can visually resemble IBD. Unfortunately, many people associate biopsies with cancer. Biopsies, however, are routinely taken in IBD-related exams as a way of providing doctors with highly specific information about the condition of the inner lining of the gastrointestinal tract. Parents and children need not feel alarmed by the prospect of a biopsy, however. Since there are no nerves to feel the pinching sensation inside the intestine, biopsies of the intestine are quick and painless.

Just as contrast studies with barium have their limitations, so, too, do endoscopic exams. Because the endoscope only examines the mucosa or innermost lining of the intestine, problems associated with Crohn's disease, particularly those involving deeper layers of the bowel, can go undetected. Likewise, biopsies can only be taken of the mucosa; this means that specific findings in the deeper layers of the bowel are sometimes overlooked. For that reason, only 10 to 15% of cases show changes on mucosal biopsy specimens that are specifically diagnostic of Crohn's disease. However, a larger percentage of biopsies will reveal inflammation suggestive of either Crohn's disease or ulcerative colitis.

TYPES OF ENDOSCOPIC EXAMS

There are different types of endoscopy. An endoscopic examination of the lower part of the colon is called a sigmoidoscopy. Colonoscopy is an endoscopic examination of the entire colon. Esophagogastroduodenoscopy is a long term often referred to by the initials EGD. This exam involves looking at the esophagus, stomach, and duodenum. Because these three areas are not commonly involved in Crohn's disease, esophagogastroduodenoscopy is not often performed in children with suspected inflammatory bowel disease.

WHERE AND HOW ENDOSCOPIC EXAMS ARE DONE

An endoscopic exam can be done in a physician's office, hospital endoscopy suite, or in an operating room. Usually these exams are done on an ambulatory basis. A child who has undergone an endoscopy is only rarely kept overnight at a hospital and is typically allowed to return home following an observation period after completion of the exam.

The anticipated cooperation of the child will be taken into account by doctors conducting the exam and the amount of sedation adjusted accordingly. When sedation is required, monitoring devices are placed on the child to ensure that heart and respiratory rates remain stable and that sufficient oxygen is being carried through the bloodstream. The child may also be provided with supplemental oxygen (via a mask-like device). Among older, less anxious children, conscious sedation with the use of such drugs as Valium®, Versed®, Demerol®, or Fentanyl® can be provided intravenously. The actual endoscopic exam can take anywhere from 15 to 60 minutes, and the patient often returns home about an hour after awakening. However, if the child is particularly anxious, completing the test may be difficult. In recent years, anesthetic agents, administered by anesthesiologists, have become available for this procedure.

PREPARATION FOR COLONOSCOPIC AND SIGMOIDOSCOPIC EXAMS

To properly view the lining of the intestine, the colon must be free of stool. A sigmoidoscopy, which is a limited endoscopic exam of the lowermost segment of the large intestine, requires somewhat less time and advance preparation than a full colonoscopic examination. Individuals usually undergo sigmoidoscopic exams after receiving an enema. However, children anxious about the procedure are sometimes given sedation to make the experience less traumatic.

For a sigmoidoscopy, the patient is positioned on a special table and a flexible tube is inserted into the rectum to provide the doctor a view of the lowermost 10 to 15 inches of the large intestine. Redness or coarseness of the surface are indicative of inflammation. There can be some bleeding of the irritated intestinal wall. Pus, which is also sometimes present, is a further indicator of the presence of inflammation and disease. When the inflammation is limited to the lowest areas of the bowel, a simple sigmoidoscopic examination may be adequate for the evaluation of ulcerative colitis. However, a simple sigmoidoscopy does not provide information about the possible activity of the disease in other regions of the colon.

A colonoscopic exam is a more extensive examination and requires a period of going without solid food, as well as the use of laxatives and special cleansing fluids. For that reason, preparations for a full colonoscopic examination must be made well ahead of time. For children, unfortunately, the preparation is often worse than the exam itself. Generally, the child must remain on clear fluids anywhere from 24 to 48 hours prior to the test and then undergo a series of enemas and laxatives. Enemas frequently are used because the colon-cleansing beverages taken by adults are usually poorly received by children, few of whom can be induced to drink unpleasant-tasting liquids.

THE COLONOSCOPY

The colonoscopy is an investigation of the entire large bowel. Since a colonoscopy involves a more extensive region than most other endoscopic exams, it should come as no surprise that a colonoscopy is a more difficult procedure, both for the child and the doctor. The endoscopist passes the instrument into the rectum to the sigmoid, from there into the descending colon, the transverse colon, the ascending colon, and all the way to the cecum. The movement of the instrument through curvatures in the colon or through inflamed areas often produces some discomfort. Occasionally, a colonoscopy may be performed all the way to the lower region of the small intestine known as the ileum. At times, colonoscopies are employed to monitor therapeutic responses to medications already being given to children. When no heavy sedation has been employed, most children will be allowed to return home following the procedure. Results, however, may need to await the interpretation of a biopsy.

TYPES OF INFLAMMATION DISCOVERED BY ENDOSCOPY

Though differences between Crohn's disease and ulcerative colitis can be subtle and are not always apparent from x-rays, when viewed through the endoscope, the two diseases often have fairly distinct appearances. Ulcerative colitis inflammation will tend to show uniform, continuous areas of inflammation. In contrast, Crohn's disease inflammation is often intermittent. Crohn's disease often "skips" over segments, leaving areas of healthy tissue between regions of inflammation. Crohn's disease also tends to be more often associated with linear ulcerations and "cobblestoning."

RISKS AND BENEFITS

When performed by trained physicians experienced in working with children, these endoscopic procedures are associated with very few risks. Although they are rare, complications from endoscopic exams do occasionally occur. For the most part, these complications tend to take the form of allergic reactions to the medications used for sedation. Allergic reactions may take the form of skin rashes, flushing of the face, and, occasionally, wheezing. These reactions are usually very brief, lasting no longer than a few minutes, and can be treated with simple medications given to treat the allergy. A serious allergic reaction in which breathing becomes difficult is managed by the administration of a medicine known to reverse the reaction. If a child proves to be allergic to a particular medication, this information should be provided to the family and the child so that the medication can be avoided in the future. It also happens on occasion that some medicines intended to sedate the child have the opposite effect and cause hyperactivity. Such a reaction, however, is not an allergy.

During the endoscopic exam, careful monitoring takes place. Medical vigilance is necessary because the drugs used to minimize discomfort and induce sleepiness in the child can also suppress the reflex to breathe, making supplemental oxygen necessary. To deal with any unusual problems, anesthesiologists trained to provide deep sedation and support for respiration can be on hand to supply the additional support occasionally required by patients with heart or lung problems. Fortunately, in actual practice, respiratory and other problems associated with these procedures are rare.

Some minor localized complications are also possible. Temporary stinging or itching at the intravenous site are among the discomforts sometimes experienced after these examinations. Following an upper endoscopy, there may be some discomfort in the throat, as well as minor gastric disturbances. After a colonoscopy, the patient will pass the gas introduced into the bowel during the test.

Other complications arising from endoscopy are rarer still. The endoscope and the biopsy instrument often used with it can cause bleeding. Such bleeding, however, is almost never significant and usually ceases spontaneously. There are endoscopic techniques designed to stop bleeding, however, and should it become necessary, bleeding can be controlled with cauterization (the application of an electrical current through the endoscope). Transfusions or surgery are rarely required for blood loss. Almost unheard of is the making of an accidental tear or hole in the wall of the bowel with the instrument. This may be serious enough to require surgery.

Fortunately, serious complications associated with these procedures are extremely rare, with an incidence of less than 1 per 1,000. Optimally, these exams make it possible for doctors to diagnose a chronic illness and begin an early and successful course of treatment.

MEDICAL DECISIONS ABOUT TESTS AND EXAMS

From a technical point of view, these endoscopic exams are fairly standard. The interpretation of medical findings, as well as the action taken after an exam, will vary according to the specialist evaluating the results. For example, specialists who treat children may differ on the role of endoscopic exams as a method of evaluating a current treatment. Repeat examinations for purposes of monitoring treatment are more common among adult IBD patients, probably because sedation is not needed by adults. The family will need to discuss with the doctor just how often these studies need to be repeated. Rarely are two or three of the same endoscopic examinations required in one year. Should a child be given a flexible sigmoidoscopy if a full colonoscopy is anticipated at some later date? This is a decision best made after full discussions with doctor, children, and parents.

While the examinations and techniques discussed in this chapter can be of great diagnostic value, the doctor is unlikely to employ them all in the treatment of a sick child. As a general matter where children are concerned, physicians will choose the particular procedure they consider most likely to yield the highest quality of diagnostic information. For example, once infectious agents have been eliminated as a cause for a child's bloody diarrhea, a colonoscopy might be reasonable. On the other hand, if a child is experiencing right-sided pain and occasional diarrhea with weight loss, and if laboratory tests are abnormal, a small bowel series might produce the highest yield.

THE UPPER ENDOSCOPY

If a patient has symptoms suggestive of Crohn's rather than ulcerative colitis, an upper endoscopy may be ordered. Symptoms of nausea, vomiting, heartburn, and pain in the upper part of the abdomen are all suggestive of a problem in the esophagus, stomach, or duodenum. An upper endoscopy may be useful in diagnosing the abnormality. In many instances, the only preparation needed for an upper endoscopy is a period of fasting. With children, doctors will often use sedation. Sometimes, to allow for a more comfortable passage of the instrument, a topical anesthetic is sprayed into the back of the mouth. The main purpose of the upper endoscopy is to look closely at the child's inflammation in an effort to determine if it is being caused by an infection, acid secretion, or Crohn's disease. Biopsied tissue studied under a microscope may be very helpful in this regard.

Another form of upper endoscopy associated with inflammatory bowel disease is endoscopic retrograde cholangiopancreaticography (ERCP). Though rarely necessary in children, at some point this exam may be required by a doctor with a need to evaluate the condition of the ducts that drain the liver and pancreas. These ducts can be blocked in IBD. In this exam, a special endoscope is passed into the duodenum, and a small tube is passed through the instrument and into the duct where bile empties from the liver, gall bladder, and pancreas. An injection of dye is made into the duct via the tube, and an x-ray is taken. This test permits an evaluation of the liver and pancreas. Scarring of the ducts that drain the liver occurs in inflammatory bowel disease, although it is unusual in the pediatric population.

SUMMARY

Many tests are available to help health care providers establish a diagnosis and identify the location of disease activity. Not all tests need to be performed in every patient with IBD. The table below summarizes some of the diagnostic tests which may be ordered.

COMMON EXAMINATIONS USED IN DIAGNOSING IBD

TYPE	PREPARATION	SEDATION	INTRAVENOUS (IV)
X-RAYS			
1. Upper GI Series	Fasting 4-8 hours	None	No
2. Barium Enema	Laxatives/Enemas	None	No
3. Abdominal Ultrasound or CT Scan	Fasting 4-8 hours Laxatives	None	Sometimes
4. KUB	None	None	No
ENDOSCOPY			
1. Esophagogastro-duodenoscopy (EGD)	Fasting 4-8 hours	Yes	Yes
2. Sigmoidoscopy	Enemas	Sometimes	Sometimes
3. Colonoscopy Laxatives/Enemas	Fasting 4-8 hours	Yes	Yes

CHAPTER 5

IS A DEFINITE DIAGNOSIS POSSIBLE?

We have discussed the barium-assisted and endoscopic examinations, as well as the biopsies which often enable a doctor to better understand and treat problems of children with inflammatory bowel disease. Here we are concerned with the location and characteristics of any discovered area of inflammation, and how location is sometimes helpful to a doctor attempting to enter a specific diagnosis of either Crohn's disease or ulcerative colitis.

TOWARD DIAGNOSTIC CERTAINTY OF CROHN'S DISEASE

The small intestine, particularly the region farthest from the stomach and closest to the large intestine (also known as the terminal ileum), is the most commonly affected area in Crohn's disease. Although often found in this ileocecal region where the large and small intestines join, Crohn's disease can occur anywhere in the gastrointestinal tract.

A discovery of inflammation in some regions of the bowel make a specific diagnosis all but certain. For example, as we have stated, ulcerative colitis is confined to the lining of the large intestine. Therefore, if it is not attributable to other causes, an area of inflammation discovered anywhere beyond the large intestine, or inflammation found deep within the walls of the bowel, indicates a child has Crohn's disease and not ulcerative colitis. If there is inflammation in the large intestine coexistent with other inflammation in the esophagus, stomach, or small intestine, once again, the disease is Crohn's. Fistulas and strictures do not occur in ulcerative colitis. Therefore, if the doctor has found evidence of these findings, the child has Crohn's disease.

DISTRIBUTION OF INFLAMMATION — CHILDREN AND ADULTS WITH CROHN'S DISEASE

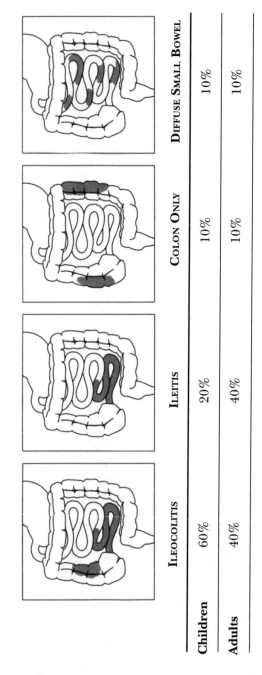

	ILEOCOLITIS	**ILEITIS**	**COLON ONLY**	**DIFFUSE SMALL BOWEL**
Children	60%	20%	10%	10%
Adults	40%	40%	10%	10%

One of the hallmarks of Crohn's disease found in biopsied tissues are granuloma formations. These formations, which do not appear in ulcerative colitis, are actually clusters of white blood cells. Unfortunately, since many of these granuloma formations are deeply imbedded in the intestinal wall, and since only the innermost lining of the intestine can be viewed or biopsied via endoscopy, granuloma formations often go undetected.

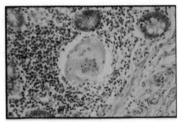

GIANT CELL

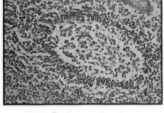

GRANULOMA

UNCERTAIN SYMPTOMS

Although Crohn's disease can occur in the large intestine, more often than not, it does not appear in the rectum. In about 10 to 15% of newly diagnosed patients, however, Crohn's disease presents only in the lining of the large intestine. In such instances, distinguishing between Crohn's and ulcerative colitis can be difficult. Nevertheless, evidence of inflammatory bowel disease in the colon which does not involve the rectum is somewhat more suggestive of Crohn's disease than ulcerative colitis.

The same type of inflammation present in ulcerative colitis, namely crypt abscesses or cryptitis, also appears in Crohn's disease. This, too, is one of several features that adds to the potential difficulty of distinguishing between the two diseases. However, if crypt abscesses are present but the area of inflammation is dispersed in different areas of the small and large intestine, the child has Crohn's disease rather than ulcerative colitis.

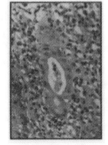

CRYPT ABSCESSES

Drawing on the above information and everything else known about the symptoms and inflammation being experienced by a child, in most instances, the doctor would now be able to enter a definitive diagnosis of either Crohn's disease or ulcerative colitis. Some doubt, however, might yet remain.

DIAGNOSTIC UNCERTAINTY

Enduring uncertainties about which of the two inflammatory bowel diseases a child is suffering from are likely to be the result of two factors: the present location or manifestation of the disease, and the limitations of the diagnostic exams available to study these diseases.

For example, at the time the child first visits the doctor, the existing IBD inflammation may be mild, subtle, or confined to the large intestine, where both diseases are sometimes diagnosed. For that reason, it may be difficult for a doctor to precisely characterize the inflammation or reach a definite diagnosis.

Although diagnostic equipment has been greatly improved over the years, at times, it still leaves something to be desired. For example, though undeniably helpful, barium-assisted exams enable a doctor to see only shapes and images, while endoscopic exams, which are also valuable, limit the doctor's view to the innermost lining of the intestine, possibly obscuring IBD symptoms embedded more deeply in the walls of the bowel.

Fortunately for the child and family, many approaches to treatment and many of the medications employed to relieve the symptoms of IBD are equally effective in treating children with ulcerative colitis or Crohn's disease. Since inflammatory bowel diseases are chronic and often brought into remission, but never healed short of surgery, over time a precise diagnosis is almost certain to be entered.

INFLAMMATION CHANGES OVER TIME

Although doctors do their best to arrest symptoms and bring them under control so a child can lead a normal life in all respects, Crohn's disease and ulcerative colitis which have been brought into full or partial remission can flare up and relapse. If, over time, an area of inflammation remains confined to the lining of the large bowel, doctors will eventually conclude that the disease is ulcerative colitis. On the other hand, if inflammation begins to spread to other regions of the bowel or to progress into the intestinal wall, the disease will eventually be diagnosed as Crohn's. Since colonoscopic exams show only the lining, not all indicators of Crohn's can be expected to show up during an initial or early endoscopic study. Linings may be inflamed, suggesting ulcerative colitis, but deeper underlying areas of disease undetected by initial biopsies may appear during subsequent examinations. When this happens, what looks, initially, like ulcerative colitis may prove in time to be Crohn's disease. Also, inflamed areas of the bowel may be initially visible only in the lining. Over time, if there occurs a thickening of the bowel wall, a diagnosis of ulcerative colitis would again be changed to one of Crohn's disease.

In ulcerative colitis, inflammatory bowel disease inflammation generally begins in the lowermost region of the large intestine known as the rectum. If only the rectum is inflamed, the child's ulcerative colitis is termed proctitis (from procto, the Latin term for rectum). Over time, ulcerative colitis can spread in an ascending fashion. When the proctitis ascends, doctors describe its extension as proctosigmoiditis. If the inflammation continues to spread upward into the transverse colon, the condition is described as left-sided ulcerative colitis. When inflammation becomes dispersed throughout the intestine, it is known as pancolitis, or total colitis.

While each of these diseases does tend to spread, Crohn's disease does not progress with the same predictability as ulcerative colitis. Crohn's often leaves patches of disease-free intestine between areas of inflammation. This phenomenon is known as "skipping." Therefore, over time, inflammation that remains confined to the large intestine and progresses in a linear fashion is likely to be diagnosed definitively as ulcerative colitis. When inflammation "skips," leaving areas of healthy bowel between regions of inflammation, the disease will come to be considered Crohn's disease.

DISTRIBUTION OF INFLAMMATION IN CHILDREN WITH ULCERATIVE COLITIS

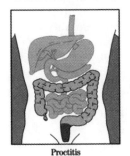
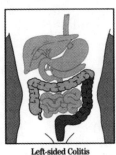
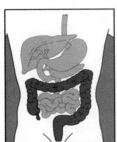

| Proctitis | Left-sided Colitis | Total Colitis (Pancolitis) |

Proctitis   Left-sided Colitis   Total Colitis

THE BEGINNING OF TREATMENT

When a child is suffering from an undiagnosed gastrointestinal disease, parents and families hope for a simple and treatable diagnosis. Some families may even believe that once a doctor makes a formal diagnosis, the child's recovery is just around the corner. Unfortunately, with Crohn's and ulcerative colitis, things are never quite that simple.

In administering the invasive exams discussed in chapter 4, doctors hope to discover information which will lead to a highly successful treatment, both in the immediate future and, since the diseases are chronic, in the years to come. Whether or not an early and definitive diagnosis is made, after completion of the required examinations, doctors will generally know enough about a child's condition to begin treatment, even if it cannot yet be said with certainty whether a child has ulcerative colitis or Crohn's disease.

For example, a child might look pale and thin and may complain of diarrhea and fever. Blood tests might have turned up evidence of anemia, and an endoscopic exam may have established inflammation as the cause of the anemia. In a child with such symptoms, treatment with a medicine containing 5-aminosalicylic acid (described in chapter 7), may be prescribed, even if the physician is uncertain whether the child has ulcerative colitis or Crohn's disease. Although a precise diagnosis may be reassuring to both the child and parents, therapy can be started and a diagnosis may become clearer in the future. Sometimes a specific finding will cause a doctor to settle on a particular treatment. For example, barium x-rays may have led to the discovery of fistulas or strictures in the small bowel. Their presence establishes a diagnosis of Crohn's, eliminates the possibility of ulcerative colitis, and may cause the physician to consider antibiotics or another form of therapy expressly intended to heal the fistula. In very many cases, however, provided the child's IBD is not severe, a precise diagnosis would be unlikely to greatly influence the form of treatment provided to children.

Children, parents, and families are well advised to remember that both ulcerative colitis and Crohn's disease can be treated with excellent success. Given proper medical care and a good response to therapy, a child can anticipate periods when gastrointestinal problems are absent and frequent appointments with the doctor are unnecessary. Although these diseases are regarded as chronic and are not presently curable, they are manageable. Someday a cure may be forthcoming. The likelihood of finding permanent cures for these diseases depends on doctors and researchers learning more about their causes. Continuing research into the immune system and chronic gastrointestinal inflammation is already beginning to produce effective new therapies.

CHAPTER 6

WHAT CAUSES INFLAMMATORY BOWEL DISEASE?

The gathering, analyzing, and synthesizing of medical information in logical and intuitive ways is the task of medical research. Research can lead to discovering the causes of disease, as well as the means by which it might be prevented. The development of new medicines useful in treating disease symptoms (aspirin for the common cold) is also the province of medical research. Sometimes, the study of a disease will lead to a means of preventing its occurrence (polio and the polio vaccine).

In searching for the causes of disease, researchers are often aided by disease demographics or population groups. Such research is known as epidemiology. Although so far, epidemiological research into inflammatory bowel disease has turned up more patterns and questions than answers, when carefully compiled and analyzed, these patterns and questions may contain clues about the cause of inflammatory bowel disease. Over time, the accumulation of research leads to an enhanced awareness of disease causes and brings about improved methods of prevention, as well as better methods of treatment.

What follows is a series of brief discussions of some promising research ideas thought to have implications for inflammatory bowel disease. Genetic factors, infectious causes, immunologic dysfunction, as well as dietary and environmental factors, all seem to be involved in the origins of IBD.

GENETICS

Inflammatory bowel disease does not appear to be inherited in the same sense that other diseases, conditions, and characteristics such as eye color are. Predisposing genetic factors do, however, seem to

increase the likelihood that certain persons will develop IBD. It is estimated, for instance, that between 20 and 40% of IBD patients have or
will have other family members with IBD. First-degree relatives of patients with Crohn's disease are about 10 times more at risk of developing the disease than members of the general population. To a lesser
extent, much the same holds true for ulcerative colitis.

A common genetic marker known as the anti-neutrophil cytoplas-
mic antibody (ANCA) appears to be a predisposing marker for patients
with ulcerative colitis. Markers, which have yet to be discovered in patients with Crohn's disease, may eventually yield important information about Crohn's. Certainly there is a good deal more that can be
learned about the role of inheritance in IBD.

Other interesting research developments touch on genetics and
the immune system. Recently published studies in this area have discussed experiments involving the elimination of certain genes from
the DNA of mice. Removal of these genes seems to create deficiencies
in mouse immune systems and produce disorders in mice that resemble
inflammatory bowel disease. These results suggest a likelihood that the
immune system is at least partially genetically influenced. When this
supposed genetic/immunologic interrelationship is altered in some way,
the immune system may become overactive, resulting in inflammation
and lesions similar to those found in inflammatory bowel disease. Normally the intestine, particularly the colon, contains a great deal of bacteria. Interestingly, the mice models did not develop inflammatory bowel
disease symptoms when their intestines were kept free of bacteria. Thus,
the development of inflammatory bowel disease may be related to an
interplay between the bacteria normally found in the intestinal tract
and an immune system affected in unknown ways by inherited factors.
This suggests that patients genetically predisposed to IBD, may develop
Crohn's disease or ulcerative colitis after being exposed to what might
be an innocuous infection to other individuals.

IMMUNOLOGIC DYSFUNCTION

The immune system is nature's way of helping the human body react
against foreign substances which should not be present in the body.
Many authorities have long suspected a connection between inflammatory bowel disease and immunologic dysfunction. For our purposes
here, the immune system response can be thought of as different types
of white blood cells dispatched by the immune system to attack foreign
proteins. Intense responses of these white blood cells lead to inflammation. In addition, other chemicals (so-called inflammatory media-
tors) are released into the tissues and cause damage, including
ulceration and swelling. This process produces the clinical picture of

inflammatory bowel disease. In ulcerative colitis, this process is confined to the tissues of the colon. In Crohn's disease the reaction is a more general response to cells lining the entire gastrointestinal tract. In addition, immune system dysfunction can affect the skin, liver, and joints, producing some of the extraintestinal symptoms (outside the gastrointestinal tract) associated with inflammatory bowel disease.

ALLERGIES

Allergies are generally caused by an immune system which overreacts to certain ingested, inhaled, or cutaneous proteins. While researchers have thus far been unable to implicate a particular food or group of foods to support the argument that inflammatory bowel disease is caused by allergic reactions to specific foods such as sugars, cereals, or milk, there are certain indications that diet plays a role in the development of inflammatory bowel disease. For example, some children and adults can be nutritionally treated for IBD with elemental formulas in which ordinary dietary protein is broken down into very small molecules. These predigested proteins seem to be much less likely to cause inflammatory reactions. This suggests that some proteins might cause reactions in the intestinal tracts of some individuals. In fact, other studies have tended to support this view. It is thought to be significant, for example, that elemental formulas can also reduce the seriousness of existing symptoms of Crohn's disease.

POSSIBLE INFECTIOUS CAUSES

Since infections of various sorts are known to cause diseases resembling IBD, for many years researchers have sought infectious agents that may actually cause Crohn's disease or inflammatory bowel disease. Recently researchers have begun pursuing the relationship between IBD and *Mycobacterium kansasii*, an organism resembling the bacteria that causes tuberculosis. This bacteria has been found to cause a disease in animals that resembles Crohn's disease. However, the medications known to eliminate these organisms in animals have not proved beneficial to individuals with inflammatory bowel disease.

Not long ago, a group of investigators found viral particles in fecal extracts of patients with inflammatory bowel disease. Another investigation has identified measles-like particles in tissues of patients with Crohn's disease. However, these findings have not been reproduced by other laboratories. Bacterial infections caused by *Salmonella, Shigella, Yersinia, Campylobacter,* and *Clostridium difficile* all produce inflammation in the intestine that resembles ulcerative colitis or Crohn's disease. Some parasites such as *Entamoeba histolytica* (amebiasis) also lead to an ulcerative colitis-like illness. In immune-deficient patients, viruses such as *Cytomegalovirus* or *Herpes virus* are also known to cause intestinal inflammation and bleeding. Occasionally, patients develop chronic IBD after an acute infection appears to initiate the disease process. However, no infection has yet been shown to cause IBD. (See table below, Diseases Resembling IBD).

DISEASES RESEMBLING IBD IN CHILDREN AND ADOLESCENTS

Infectious Causes:

Mycobacterium Tuberculosis
Salmonella
Shigella
Campylobacter
Yersinia
Clostridium difficile
Entamoeba histolytica
Enteropathic Escherichia coli (0157:H7)
Rotavirus
Cytomegalovirus

Noninfectious Causes:

Allergic (Protein-induced) colitis
Gluten enteropathy
Lymphoma

ENVIRONMENT

Several studies have looked at environmental factors which may predispose individuals to develop Crohn's disease. At one time or another, refined sugar, margarine, and alcohol were all suspected of predisposing some people to develop Crohn's. However, no study has yet demonstrated that any specific food definitely causes or predisposes a person to develop this disease. A study done in Israel of a large number of children with IBD investigated possible connections between inflammatory bowel disease and life experience. The study found no relationship to inflammatory bowel disease and birth order, number of siblings, or early diet (cereal, formula versus breast feeding). Nor was any correlation found between inflammatory bowel disease and any other environmental factors. Although there have been clusters of outbreaks of IBD in neighborhoods, these occurrences have remained rare, and efforts to find a reason for such clustering have so far been unsuccessful.

STRESS

Studies seeking to evaluate the role played by stress in IBD have been inconclusive. However, there are indications that under conditions of stress, IBD patients may notice their symptoms more, or have more difficulty coping with relapses of disease symptoms. In fact, these relapses tend to occur when children or teens with IBD are under unusual amounts of stress. In adolescence, these periods tend to coincide with the beginning of the school year. Tensions regarding homework or examinations are also suspected of sometimes triggering or exacerbating IBD symptoms. Along these same lines, unpleasant job situations or the stresses of family life tend to make IBD symptoms more troublesome for adults. Although stress does not cause IBD, it can readily affect how a child or adult deals with symptoms of the disease.

CIGARETTES

Epidemiological studies have found that fewer smokers seem to develop ulcerative colitis than nonsmokers, a finding which apparently gave rise to an experimental effort to treat ulcerative colitis patients with supplementary nicotine patches. This particular study seems to contradict the findings of another study suggesting that passive smoking may predispose children to Crohn's disease and ulcerative colitis. Further investigation will undoubtedly be needed before many doctors begin prescribing nicotine patches for patients with ulcerative colitis. In fact, patients with inflammatory bowel disease who were treated with nicotine patches experienced many side effects from wearing them. Also, unfortunately for smokers looking for good news, other studies have shown that smokers develop Crohn's disease more frequently than nonsmokers.

COMBINATIONS OF CAUSES

Infectious agents, genetics, and the immune system all seem to interact in some way with environmental factors in producing these diseases. Unraveling the interactions of these potentially contributing factors is difficult and confusing. Children bothered by inflammatory bowel disease symptoms at certain times of the year should suspect environmental allergies as acting like triggers. Similarly, certain foods or stressful events that seem to cause a child to experience increased symptoms should, to the extent possible, be avoided or reduced whenever possible. Individual decisions to avoid certain foods or beverages, however, should be discussed with a physician.

PART II

TREATMENT OF INFLAMMATORY BOWEL DISEASE

CHAPTER 7

THE TREATMENT OF CHILDREN

Understandably, families want to believe the "right" drug will cure a child's inflammatory bowel disease in much the way penicillin alleviates strep throat. Unfortunately, with IBD, things do not happen that way. No "miracle drug" permanently alleviates symptoms and eradicates these illnesses. Crohn's disease is a chronic disease with no known cure, while ulcerative colitis is a chronic disease with no cure short of major surgery.

The good news is that while many people associate inflammatory bowel disease with hospitalization, absence from school, surgery, missed work, and unremitting pain, the fact is, most people with IBD lead ordinary lives and never enter the hospital.

Just as the symptoms of these diseases are complex and the sites of inflammation various, so are the forms of treatment provided to a child with IBD. Many good medications bring about symptomatic relief and remission in children and adults with IBD, and research into the development of still more effective medicines goes on each day. But, until the time comes when research provides a way to prevent or cure inflammatory bowel disease, children, parents, and doctors will necessarily continue to work with a variety of imperfect medicines, all of them capable of providing relief, and all of them capable of producing side effects.

The potential benefits to children of the medicines described in this chapter are enormous. Potent medicines, however, may produce side effects. Children taking these medicines must be carefully monitored. Medicines producing side effects without conferring health benefits will be probably be discontinued by the doctor. On the other hand, not all side effects are serious, and there are instances in which patients, doctors, and parents are willing to endure some minor side effects in order to obtain the symptom-reducing benefits of particular medicines.

Under ideal circumstances, your child will be provided with a form of medical treatment that effectively reduces IBD symptoms and produces no side effects. But the relief can be all too temporary. It is a particularly distressing fact of life with inflammatory bowel disease that symptoms once brought into remission, thanks to a particular medication, may return full force when the medication is reduced or withdrawn. Among children, families, and doctors, this particular frustration has been known to give rise to a sense that IBD symptoms come and go without much respect for the medicines prescribed to alleviate them. It sometimes seems that the best that modern medicine can do is to fight inflammatory bowel disease symptoms until they subside on their own.

As a rule, a physician attempts to provide a child with the most effective drug associated with the mildest possible side effects. Less potent medications with fewer side effects are prescribed for children whose symptoms are mild, while the more powerful medicines with potentially stronger side effects are reserved for those with more dramatic symptoms.

THE HOPE OF INSTANT RELIEF

While aspirin can often relieve a headache in an hour, and an antibiotic can clear up an ear infection in a few days, the medications taken for inflammatory bowel disease tend to work more slowly. It may be weeks or months before it becomes apparent whether or not a particular drug is going to have a beneficial effect on a child's disease. Even after a medication begins to be effective, children are still likely to experience some episodes of pain and discomfort. For these reasons, it is best, though admittedly difficult, for children and families to cultivate an attitude of patience, doing all they can to remain optimistic and hopeful. Disappointment, slow progress, and an apparent lack of results are a part of the picture. So too are successes. Just as formerly effective medicines sometimes cease to bring symptomatic relief, the reverse also happens. Sometimes a medicine that showed no sign of having an impact against a child's disease, suddenly begins to have a beneficial effect.

TOPICAL AND SYSTEMIC MEDICINES

Topical medicines are those which work directly on injured tissues. An ointment applied to sunburn, for example, would be considered a topical medication. To this explanation should be added, however, that even medications taken by mouth can be considered topical medicines, provided they do not principally cross into the blood stream, and provided they have a direct effect on the lining of the bowel. Whenever appropriate, doctors tend to prefer topical medications to the systemic medicines absorbed into the body. This is particularly true in inflammatory bowel disease, because topical medicines often relieve a child's symptoms with fewer side effects and complications. Since they are applied directly to the inflamed anal or rectal tissue, suppositories or special enemas are considered topical medications. Often, these topical preparations are effective in reducing inflammation and soreness in the lower colon.

MEDICATIONS CONTAINING 5-AMINOSALICYLIC ACID

After World War II, it became apparent that sulfasalazine, a drug used to treat rheumatoid arthritis, was also quite effective in eliminating or reducing the gastrointestinal inflammation of inflammatory bowel disease.

Sulfasalazine, which is sometimes known by its brand name, Azulfidine®, is made up of two components broken down by numerous bacteria in the lower intestine. One of the components, 5-aminosalicylic acid (5-ASA), is an anti-inflammatory agent (similar to aspirin) that blocks some of the chemical by-products of inflammatory cells. The anti-inflammatory properties of the medication come into play when the 5-ASA portion of the medication comes into contact with the diseased lining of the intestine. The other 5-ASA component is a sulfa-type antibiotic important in transporting and distributing it throughout the colon. Without the sulfa element to disperse its anti-inflammatory properties, 5-ASA would be absorbed in the small bowel and fail to reach the region of inflammation to which it was being directed. Therefore, although the drug is taken orally, sulfasalazine can be thought of as a topical treatment because of the way it is distributed.

The side effects caused by either component of this drug include nausea, headaches, a ringing in the ears, and a decreased sperm count. Less frequently, 5-ASA is associated with damage to the bone marrow, liver, and even the pancreas. Since heavy initial dosages can meet with poor results and trigger side effects, doctors often gradually increase dosage of this medicine over a period of several days.

Rashes are among sulfasalazine's most serious undesirable side effects. The sulfasalazine rash, which occurs in 10 to 20% of patients, typically appears as a red, fine, bumpy inflammation over much of the body. Since this drug's more serious systemic reactions frequently follow the appearance of this rash, it is very important for the child to discontinue taking sulfasalazine after a rash becomes visible.

Though it may have some beneficial effect on inflammation of the small intestine in Crohn's disease, sulfasalazine is most effective in the large intestine, where the bond between its antibiotic and anti-inflammatory components is broken down. Provided that about two weeks are allowed for the drug to take full effect, sulfasalazine may reduce symptoms in mild to moderate ulcerative colitis, and even become the primary treatment provided to some IBD patients. The major problem with sulfasalazine is that it always remains a topical treatment and may not reduce the Crohn's disease inflammations located beyond the intestinal lining, deeper in the walls of the bowel.

In instances where it is effective, sulfasalazine has prophylactic or preventive benefits as well. Several reports have shown that ongoing maintenance on sulfasalazine reduces the episodic flare-ups of ulcerative colitis. In addition, in left-sided or distal disease, the use of sulfasalazine is thought to decrease the likelihood that ulcerative colitis will spread to the proximal large intestine.

The serious side effects triggered by the sulfa component of sulfasalazine have given rise to a search for a drug containing only 5-ASA. Unfortunately, it has been discovered that when 5-ASA is given by itself, the drug is often absorbed before it reaches the inflamed area. When two different 5-ASA components are linked together, they form a new compound that is poorly absorbed in the upper bowel and eventually reaches the distal bowel. This compound, olsalazine or Dipentum®, eventually reaches the distal bowel where it separates into the two 5-ASA components of sulfasalazine. While initially thought to be of great benefit, Dipentum® is actually no more effective than sulfasalazine. However, olsalazine is often useful to children who have experienced side effects from the sulfa component of sulfasalazine. Although many children tolerate olsalazine without difficulty, olsalazine is known to cause more diarrhea than sulfasalazine.

Other 5-ASA preparations, such as mesalamine, have become available in recent years with an acrylic (Asacol®) or a cellulose (Pentasa®) coating. These coatings are provided in an effort to minimize the amount of the medication released in the stomach and upper GI tract in order to deliver most of the medication to the small intestine. However, despite these coatings, there still appears to be significant systemic absorption and, unfortunately, many children intolerant of sulfasalazine have similar problems with Asacol® and Pentasa®. On the other hand, since these latter drugs do seem to be released more proximally in the small intestine, they may be more effective than sulfasalazine in the treatment of Crohn's disease. Some experts believe these drugs can even prevent recurrences of Crohn's disease. A multicenter study to evaluate this claim is currently under way.

Lastly, mesalamine can be administered rectally, either as an enema or in suppository form, in a preparation marketed as Rowasa®. This medication is used in patients with distal disease and in patients who may also be on other medicines but who still get tenesmus or anal spasms. Although many children do not like enemas or suppositories, when used appropriately, they can be very beneficial.

ANTIBIOTICS

That antibiotics can significantly reduce the gastrointestinal inflammation associated with Crohn's disease is clear. Since antibiotics are primarily used to combat bacterial infections, why they should have an alleviating effect on the symptoms of children with inflammatory bowel disease is not well understood. Speculation is that some of the inflammatory processes of Crohn's disease and ulcerative colitis are mediated or exacerbated by bacteria, which when reduced, bring about symptomatic improvements in a child's IBD. While not all children respond positively to antibiotics, many do. And compared with other forms of intervention such as steroids, antibiotics are better tolerated and seem to produce fewer side effects. Typical antibiotics used include metronidazole, cephalexin, tetracycline (older children), ciprofloxacillin (older children only) and metronidazole. Antibiotics are also used to treat intra-abdominal abscesses and fistulas, which are abnormal connections between loops of bowel or between bowel and skin.

METRONIDAZOLE

Metronidazole seems particularly helpful in treating perirectal disease and fistulas, but may reduce inflammation as well. Like any medication, however, metronidazole produces side effects in some children. These include numbness, prickling, and tingling sensations. Episodes of nausea, furry tongue, and a lingering metallic taste in the mouth are also reported. Individuals who consume alcohol while taking metronidazole may experience severe nausea and vomiting.

CORTICOSTEROIDS

Corticosteroids were first introduced into the treatment of inflammatory bowel disease during the late 1950s, prior to which patient mortality rates were high, and operations not altogether successful. Because corticosteroids were so effective in providing patient relief, there followed a period of time when they were used in treating IBD to the exclusion of almost all other medications and forms of treatment. Eventually, this indiscriminate use led to the understanding that while steroids relieve many IBD symptoms, they are also capable of producing some long-lasting and potent side effects. These days, steroids are still regarded as an effective form of treatment. However, their usage is more carefully monitored and their side effects followed closely.

For many, the term steroids evokes images of the muscle-building androgen steroids frequently abused by athletes. In fact, the steroids used in inflammatory bowel disease are not the same as those used by body builders. The corticosteroids used in IBD are a class of hormones naturally produced by the adrenal glands to control the body's reaction to stress, blood pressure, sugar levels, and to regulate inflammation. When used for pharmaceutical purposes, these synthetic steroids are usually administered in high dosages and can dramatically reduce IBD-related inflammation.

For sick children who are often absent from school or missing out on social life, steroids can be very effective in providing relief, often enabling a child to return to normal activities. However, with their use come significant side effects. Fortunately, many of the side effects of corticosteroids are short-lived and disappear once steroids are withdrawn. If taken over a long period of time, however, they can give rise to more serious and enduring side effects.

SIDE EFFECTS OF STEROIDS

SHORT TERM	LONG TERM
Increased Appetite	Poor Wound Healing
Stomach Irritations	Muscle Weakness
Nausea/Vomiting	"Stretch" Marks
Insomnia	Increased Blood Sugar
Headache	Irregular Menstruation
Dizziness	Delayed Growth
High Blood Pressure	Weak Bones
Night Sweats	Increased Hair
Fluid Retention	Cataracts
	Acne
	Susceptibility to Infection

The cosmetic side effects of steroids, generally reversed when they are discontinued, include a Cushingnoid appearance characterized by a swelling of the face, a loss of muscle in the arms and legs, and increased fat in the abdomen and chest. Other common side effects include acne, stretch marks, fluid retention, and increased body hair, all especially troubling to most adolescents. In addition, short-term steroid use can lead to irritation of the stomach, increases in blood pressure, and a diabetes-like condition. The increased pressures steroids create within the central nervous system are sometimes manifested as headaches, mood changes, or sleep disturbances. In many instances, reduced dosages alleviate these side effects.

The more serious and enduring side effects associated with steroids are brought on by long-term use. These side effects include a loss of minerals from bones, a susceptibility to compression fractures of bones, inflammation or destruction of specific joint spaces, interference with physical growth, and cataracts.

The most common steroid preparation, prednisone, is typically given initially at a high dose, then gradually reduced in dosage once inflammation is brought under control. An important side effect of prednisone is that it puts the adrenal glands "to sleep." These glands can sense if there is cortisone or, its synthetic equivalent, prednisone, in the blood stream. When prednisone is taken every day, the adrenal glands will respond by shutting down the production of cortisone. Once shut down, the adrenal glands are slow to resume natural production of cortisone again. Consequently, prednisone therapy must be reduced gradually. In this regard, it is important to notify the doctor if a child taking prednisone develops infections, needs surgery or dental work, or is involved in a serious accident. These unusual stresses to the system may require temporary increases in prednisone therapy. These events would normally stimulate the adrenal gland to produce more steroid, which it is incapable of doing when the gland's function has been depressed by synthetic steroids.

In some cases, steroids are prescribed rectally in the form of enemas or foams. By providing topical steroid preparations rather than orally ingested steroids, doctors hope for localized results with minimal side effects. Because rectal dosages of steroids are still distributed to the blood stream at 25% of the levels of orally administered steroids, even rectally administered steroids provide no guarantee the child will avoid the Cushingnoid side effects associated with these drugs. Medications can still be absorbed into the bloodstream through the lining of the rectum, or even through the skin.

It can be as much as a week before the anti-inflammatory effects of steroids begin to have an effect on symptoms. Regrettably, it is often not until the child begins to show some of the Cushingnoid side effects that a therapeutic response to the intestinal inflammation becomes apparent. Steroids can be provided intravenously to patients sick enough to require hospitalization. But, except in urgent cases, doctors often prefer to give a patient a trial of oral steroids before administering them intravenously. Specialists often debate the best methods of introducing steroids into the system, though there seems to be very little documentation to justify all the differences of opinion. In all likelihood, the methods of introduction are probably equally effective. However, it is important to recognize that different steroids, whether administered orally or rectally, will have different potencies and may result in different side effects.

Though not yet available in the United States, budesonide, the latest topical steroid, has shown great benefit in initial trials. Although it, too, can be administered rectally, this medication seems to be more effective when taken orally. Such a method allows it to topically treat Crohn's disease inflammation in the small intestine. Significantly, because budesonide tends to be more quickly metabolized than prednisone, its side effects seem to be fewer and milder than many of those associated with prednisone and other commonly used steroids.

THE LIMITATIONS OF STEROIDS

The major problem with the use of steroids for these illnesses, is that inflammatory bowel disease symptoms may still be present or return after they are withdrawn. Since inflammation can return and prolonged steroid usage can be a significant problem, the medical options in such instances consist of reintroducing steroids, or trying some other unproven form of medication. Since side effects from steroids are cumulative and worsen over time, most physicians will tend to seek another form of treatment for the steroid-dependent child.

ABOUT IMMUNOSUPPRESSIVE AGENTS

As has been mentioned, there is a widely held and at least partly justifiable view that inflammatory bowel disease results in whole or part from a failure of the activated immune system to shut itself down. To simplify the argument somewhat, the immune system of children with IBD tends to overreact to some unknown stimuli by producing an overabundance of inflammatory cells, resulting in inflammation of the gastrointestinal tract. Supporting this view is evidence that inflammation and other IBD symptoms can be reduced or alleviated by slowing down or suppressing the overly responsive immune system. The most common medications used to suppress the immune system are 6-mercaptopurine and azathioprine. Cyclosporine and methotrexate may also be provided. Over the last ten or fifteen years, these medications have been used to treat children with severe inflammation who cannot discontinue steroid use without experiencing a flare-up of disease symptoms.

Unfortunately, immunosuppressive agents, too, produce side effects. Even when it is not immediately obvious they are doing so, these drugs suppress the immune system. In the process, they render children potentially more susceptible to viral and bacterial infections. There is, for example, a very real concern about young people who are taking immunosuppressive agents contracting routine viral infections such as chicken pox. Because of this concern, immunosuppressive drugs bring risks which are not always acceptable in the treatment of children. More importantly, since healthy immune systems seem to thwart the development of malignant cells, children and other patients with suppressed immune systems may face slightly increased risks of developing cancer, particularly lymphoma. Although no one has ever proven an increased malignancy rate in IBD children treated with immunosuppressive drugs, these at least theoretical concerns must be considered before introducing them to a child.

In addition to the fact that they render immune systems vulnerable, immunosuppressives have been associated with possible damage to bone marrow. For that reason, children taking immunosuppressives require frequent blood counts to ensure that the bone marrow is producing blood cells (a discussion of blood tests is found in chapter 3). Fortunately bone marrow problems are usually reversed when immunosuppressive use is discontinued. Mouth ulcerations and inflammation of the pancreas and liver have also been associated with these agents.

Despite the risks associated with the use of immunosupressives, medically informed adults may decide in favor of immunosuppressive treat-

Shortly before my sixteenth birthday I began to notice blood in my stools. I was afraid, but I didn't tell my parents because I thought that I might have done something wrong, and that maybe it would go away. But in the fall of that year, when I started my sophomore year in high school, I was diagnosed as having ulcerative colitis. It was a frightening time of embarrassment and uncertainty. Embarrassment, because I was afraid to go anywhere for fear of being too far from a bathroom; and uncertainty, because no matter what we tried we could not bring my condition into remission. I was up to 40 mg of prednisone per day and felt fat and foolish looking. Even experimental drugs proved to be no help. Finally I was presented with the option of surgery, which I am very thankful I accepted. I had tremendous confidence in my physicians and I now lead a very normal life. Had I waited longer to opt for the surgery, or not made that decision, the outcome would have been very different. Finally, I would like to say that keeping a positive outlook and maintaining a sense of humor will go along way in helping you through the process.

—ANDREW

ment in the hope of obtaining symptomatic relief from inflammatory bowel disease symptoms. But families should be cautious where children are concerned. Young people suffering from severe ulcerative colitis considered to be either steroid dependent or steroid refractory, may be better directed toward surgery, thereby alleviating the disease and avoiding the risks associated with taking immunosuppressives. Young people with severely steroid-dependent or steroid-refractory Crohn's disease, however, face significantly different decisions. Since surgery in Crohn's disease rarely brings about enduring results, immunosuppressive agents may offer young people with Crohn's disease benefits outweighing the risks of immunosuppressive therapy.

While there are potential unknown risks associated with long-term immunosuppressive use, these drugs have been shown to provide some individuals with significant benefits. Along with freeing steroid-dependent children from the risks and side effects of steroids, they have been shown to induce growth in children whose physical maturity has been slowed by severe IBD. Further, they have proven very effective in closing fistulas.

The fistula-healing properties of these medicines (as well as their other potential benefits) may not begin to make themselves felt for two or three months after they have been introduced into the system, however. For this reason, children taking steroids for symptomatic relief may have to continue with them until the immunosuppressive agents begin to take effect. In such cases, results can be monitored by lab tests.

Although doctors remain cautious about immunosuppressive drugs for a child who might receive equal or nearly equal benefit from other medical options, it is perhaps significant that there now exists a 20-year history with these drugs. So far, at least, there does not appear to be an increase in cancer in individuals who have used immunosuppressives.

CYCLOSPORINE

Cyclosporine, which initially made liver transplantation possible, is one of the more hotly debated immunosuppressive drugs used in the treatment of inflammatory bowel disease. In addition to its value to some ulcerative colitis patients, cyclosporine has also been shown to be effective in treating symptoms of Crohn's disease. Cyclosporine begins to work more quickly than other immunosuppressive drugs. For that reason, it may be given as a treatment of last resort when surgery appears imminent for seriously ill patients with ulcerative colitis. Some authorities, however, believe that cyclosporine merely postpones the inevitable need for surgery, all the while placing the child at risk of developing side effects which include those already discussed for

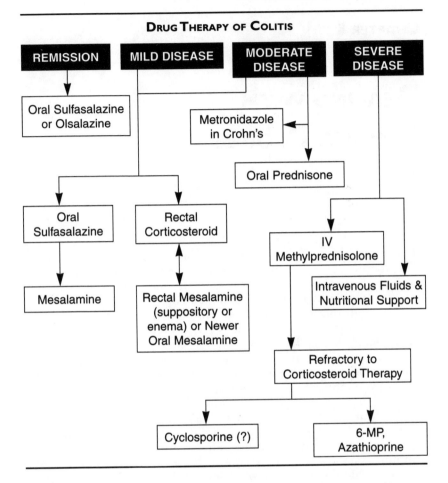

DRUG THERAPY OF COLITIS

immunosuppressives, as well as hypertension, kidney injury, seizures, and hirsutism (the appearance of unwanted body hair).

METHOTREXATE

Methotrexate has been used in the treatment of adult patients. Occasionally it has been provided to children who have developed toxic reactions to some of the more commonly used steroids. Methotrexate is generally administered intramuscularly only until another more effective medication can be found. The most serious side effect associated with methotrexate is injury to the liver.

CHAPTER 8

DEALING WITH
SPECIFIC PROBLEMS

A general discussion of common inflammatory bowel disease symptoms is found in chapter 2, which provides an overview of symptoms. Our particular focus here is on the subtlety, significance, and likely treatments of highly specific IBD symptoms and their complications.

Although there is currently no cure for Crohn's disease and surgery is the only permanent remedy for ulcerative colitis, a child with inflammatory bowel disease is in no way condemned to a life of pain and discomfort. It should be emphasized that uncounted numbers of inflammatory bowel disease patients respond well to medical treatments and live very normal lives. Inconvenienced at times, these individuals do not, as a group, consider themselves disabled or debilitated.

Medical care, in which parents, children, and young adults play an increasing role, can provide abiding relief and many years of remission to most children and adults with inflammatory bowel disease. While symptoms vary and there is no typical course of treatment for IBD, it is fair to say that the symptoms of children will respond favorably to the medical treatment they do receive.

Once progress is made in alleviating a child's symptoms, the child and family may want to eliminate medications in the hope of being free of the side effects, risks, inconveniences, and expenses associated with their use. More experienced in the treatment of these diseases, however, the doctor is likely to want to maintain the child on reduced dosages of medicines that seem to have produced an overall improvement.

While some remissions of inflammatory bowel disease symptoms are more complete and enduring than others, even under the best of circumstances, various gastrointestinal symptoms will recur from time to time. Such symptoms might take the form of renewed outbreaks of old symptoms, or "new" symptoms may appear — new in the sense of being unprecedented in a particular child's experience.

For the doctor, the first order of business will be to learn if these latest symptoms are IBD-related. It is important for children and parents to remember that intercurrent infectious illnesses such as viral gastroenteritis or flu-like symptoms strike all children from time to time. If a child feels unwell, it may be reassuring to know that another family member is ill or that a "stomach flu" is making the rounds at school.

Until these new or renewed symptoms can be evaluated, the doctor may be reluctant to radically depart from the medical treatments that have effected an improvement in the child. Newly introduced medicines could restimulate inflammatory bowel disease symptoms or otherwise disrupt the child's improved health. Over-the-counter medicines commonly taken to relieve aches, pains, and flu symptoms could relieve these new symptoms yet bring on a new round of inflammatory bowel symptoms. For these reasons, confronted by new symptoms that might or might not be IBD-related, the doctor may believe the first and best course of action is no action at all. Patience and fortitude may be in order.

Such decisions, of course, will necessarily be made on an individual basis. Under some circumstances, the doctor may consider recommending a particular over-the-counter medication deemed unlikely to interfere with the actions of IBD medicines already being provided. Some of these non-prescription medications can be of great benefit, while others are likely to have undesirable side effects. Check with the child's doctor if there are unexpected symptoms.

If a child's new or exacerbated symptoms *do* turn out to be caused by inflammatory bowel disease, the doctor, patient, and family, will have to decide together about the advisability of seeking a new course of treatment or simply increasing the dosages of medications already being taken. These decisions, of course, will depend on the specific symptoms being experienced.

ABDOMINAL PAIN

Abdominal pain in the right lower quadrant is likely to be due to underlying Crohn's disease. In contrast, pain associated with ulcerative colitis, which tends to be relieved by defecation, often takes the form of cramps in the left lower quadrant of the abdomen. Mid-epigastric pain is often indicative of acid peptic disease. Some IBD patients regularly take medications that predispose them to ulcers or ulcer-like conditions. Crohn's disease is associated with these ulcer-type conditions in up to 50% of patients. When a child experiences abdominal pain, a gastrointestinal endoscopy will sometimes reveal a clinically treatable ulcer-like inflammation. Reluctant to immediately order an invasive endoscopic exam, the doctor may instead choose to provide a trial of anti-ulcer therapy and observe the child's response. However, when the stomach or upper intestine seem to be involved, an upper endoscopy may be necessary and may enable the doctor to distinguish a Crohn's disease inflammation from acid-related problems.

If abdominal pain is accompanied by diarrhea, the passing of gas, or cramps, the problem may be acquired lactose intolerance. When warranted, a lactose intolerance test can be performed by collecting breath samples after a child has swallowed a large dose of lactose, the sugar in milk. In lactose intolerance, intestinal bacteria will digest the lactose your child is unable to tolerate, and doctors will be able to detect a measurable increase of hydrogen in the child's exhaled breaths. Avoiding lactose-containing foods and beverages may provide the child with abdominal pain relief until such a test can be administered. But parents should be aware, in this regard, that lactose-free diets may require supplementary calcium.

Under the careful supervision of a physician, and along with dietary counseling, small amounts of fiber may be introduced into the child's diet. However, some children with IBD can be made worse by adding bran to their diets. Therefore, if at all, bran should be introduced in low doses. As with the addition of any dietary fiber, extra water must be consumed daily in order for the fiber to be properly utilized. Ask your doctor how much additional water is necessary.

RECTAL BLEEDING

Rectal bleeding is definitely a symptom of some concern in inflammatory bowel disease and its appearance should always be evaluated by a physician. Although any amount of blood in the toilet is alarming, there may be less of it than there initially appears to be. Even so, rectal bleeding usually signals inflammation of the colon. Children with limited distal disease, namely inflammation of the rectum only, can experience isolated rectal bleeding, abdominal pain, or diarrhea. These children may experience a sense of urgency accompanied by an inability to retain stool. Alternatively, they may feel an urge to pass stool without managing to do so. In either instance, rectally administered 5-ASA in the form of Rowasa® suppositories or enemas can often control these symptoms and forestall the need for corticosteroids. Steroids can also be provided rectally, in the form of foams, suppositories, or enemas. If rectal bleeding is persistent, a complete blood count (CBC) should be obtained to ensure that an anemia is not developing. If bleeding continues after rectally instituted steroids have been introduced, it generally means that the inflamed area is not responding to treatment. This occurs when the provided medication is ineffective or an inflammation is beyond reach of the suppository, enema, or foam. Under some circumstances, an endoscopic exam may lead to a better understanding of the child's condition and a more effective form of therapy.

ANEMIA

A child with fatigue, lack of energy, and a pale or sallow appearance may be anemic. Anemia is quite common in IBD, usually attributable to secondary iron deficiency stemming from chronic, slow, gastrointestinal blood loss. However, an examination of the shape of the red blood cells and blood count may suggest other causes. A review of the child's nutritional history, along with an evaluation of the therapy the child has been receiving, is important. Since sulfasalazine is known to interfere with folate absorption, folic acid is always provided to children taking sulfasalazine. Ileal disease or an ileal resection may result in poor absorption of vitamin B-12, causing anemia. Anorexia, or a lack of appetite, may also contribute to nutritional anemias. If a child's anemia symptoms are relatively mild, iron in the form of pills or liquid may be beneficial. Unfortunately, supplementary iron causes occasional abdominal cramps. Vitamin B-12 deficiency is rare, but when it occurs, intramuscular injections every one to three months are required. Injections of such frequency are necessary because vitamin B-12 may not be absorbed well, particularly by patients who have active disease of the rectum or those who have undergone surgical resections.

DIARRHEA

Children with diarrhea have loose, watery bowel movements. Semi-formed stool is the consistency of pudding, but actual diarrhea can be poured. Cultures of the stool may help the doctor discover if the child's diarrhea is related to inflammatory bowel disease or stems from an infection. In IBD-related diarrhea, increases in the medication given to reduce bowel inflammation usually result in improvement. If the diarrhea persists, a change of primary treatment may be necessary. Higher doses of a medication already in use, a different combination of medications, or a trial of an entirely new medication could bring about the desired result. If extensive regions of the small bowel have been affected by Crohn's disease or resected via surgery, a generalized malabsorptive condition can cause chronic diarrhea. In such instances, a special diet may be required. Ordinarily, bile produced in the liver enters the upper end of the small intestine and is reabsorbed or taken up at the end of the small intestine. However, if this part of the bowel has been surgically removed (ileal resection) or is inflamed (ileitis), bile salts may not be absorbed and instead go into the colon, causing irritation and diarrhea. Such a condition may respond to cholestyramine therapy, a binding of the bile salts.

A trial of anti-diarrheal medications may be of some use, but a word of caution is necessary. Even though many of these remedies can be purchased over-the-counter, they may predispose a patient to develop toxic megacolon. Toxic megacolon is a condition where the large intestine becomes dilated and the patient is very sick. Anti-diarrheal medication should, therefore, be used by those with inflammatory bowel disease *only* when prescribed by a physician.

FATIGUE

Ensuring that teenagers with inflammatory bowel disease get enough sleep is important. Family decisions about extra-curricular activities such as soccer practice may have to be reevaluated if a child occasionally complains of fatigue. However, persistent fatigue should be brought to the attention of the doctor. Fatigue may indicate resurgent disease activity and, in fact, may be the only symptom of an exacerbation of IBD. Dietary habits should be studied and tests conducted for specific nutrient deficiencies such as iron or vitamin B-12. Depression, discussed in later chapters of this book, is also closely associated with fatigue. A review of the patient's recent social history, relationships, and self-esteem may show a child who could benefit from psychological counseling.

FEVER

Frequent fevers or fevers lasting longer than 48 hours may signal the presence of disease activity. Oral antipyretics, medications that lower fevers, like acetaminophen, may be used to reduce fevers as needed. But these should not be taken for prolonged periods of time. Fever may also indicate the onset of a complication, such as a fistula or abscess. A careful evaluation of such possibilities is important.

LOSS OF APPETITE

When eating causes abdominal pain or a feeling of fullness, some children gradually lose interest in food. In young people with Crohn's disease, loss of appetite is often an indication of disease activity requiring medical attention. A dietary history, laboratory studies, even x-rays or endoscopic studies may be necessary. Depression should also be considered as a possible cause of diminished appetite. So-called appetite stimulants have no proven role in effectively dealing with the loss of appetite experienced by some children with IBD.

WEIGHT LOSS

Weight loss is another indicator of disease activity, especially in patients with Crohn's disease. Decreased caloric intake resulting from loss of appetite is the usual reason for weight loss, but sometimes food may be incompletely absorbed, contributing to the problem. There is an important difference between a failure to gain weight and actual weight loss. The latter can be a symptom of more serious complications. A medical evaluation, together with an attempt to discover the underlying reasons for weight loss are necessary.

GROWTH DELAY

Undernutrition, active disease, or steroid medications can stunt growth. Fortunately, when taken on an every other day basis, reduced dosages of steroids often produce the desirable medical results without inducing significant growth delays. However, since undertreatment and continued disease activity are commonly the cause of slowed growth, a nutritional evaluation, coupled with supplementation or even nasogastric feedings, may be indicated. Children and parents should be presented with options and alternatives and encouraged to become more involved in any new form of therapy intended to address this problem.

DELAYED MATURATION AND SEXUAL GROWTH

Delayed maturation or retarded sexual development are often indications of chronic disease activity. Again, appropriate nutritional therapy and the subsequent reduction of inflammatory symptoms will ordinarily bring about renewed physical development.

EXTRAINTESTINAL SYMPTOMS

Most extraintestinal manifestations seem to result from inflammatory problems or a resurgence of disease activity in the bowel. The most common extraintestinal manifestations are mouth sores and joint pains. From time to time, both of these problems will occur in up to 20% of patients. Although mouth sores can interfere with eating, they usually disappear and are more of an annoyance than anything else. Topical mouth washes with local anesthetics can be of some benefit until they do. Altering the child's therapeutic regimen may be the answer.

In contrast, joint symptoms can be quite troublesome, the more so since they tend to restrict a child's activities and occur at times when gastrointestinal symptoms are otherwise quiet. In instances where bowel symptoms have been reduced, doctors may be reluctant to order increases in overall therapy and may want to temporize with non-steroidal anti-inflammatory drugs such as those containing ibuprofen. Overuse of ibuprofen, however, can be more harmful than beneficial. Physical therapy for joint pain has also been tried in some patients. Fortunately, arthritis in children with IBD almost never causes chronic damage to the joint spaces.

Erythema nodosum and *Pyoderma gangrenosum* are relatively rare skin lesions found in inflammatory bowel disease patients, occurring in no more than 1 in 25 adult patients and probably less frequently in children. *Erythema nodosum* takes the form of raised red nodules on the lower front portion of the legs and resemble mosquito bites. *Pyoderma gangrenosum* are small pus-filled lesions, usually found on the hands and feet. Naturally, both types of lesions can cause parents concern until they are properly identified and treated. Occasionally they are treated by local injections of steroids, but both generally respond to increases in the therapy provided for the bowel symptoms.

THE EYES

Various inflammations of the eye occur in some individuals with inflammatory bowel disease. The most common of these are uveitis, episcleritis, and iritis. Sensitivity to light, tearing, and pain are the common symptoms of these ophthalmological conditions. Treatment usually consists of topical drops. Ophthalmologists should examine children with IBD yearly for signs of inflammation, and special care should be taken with children whose steroid use might produce side effects leading to cataracts.

LIVER-AND-KIDNEY-RELATED COMPLICATIONS

About 3% of children with IBD develop inflammation of the liver or ducts outside the liver. The pancreas, the digestive gland adjacent to the liver, is sometimes involved as well. Although under rare circumstances, liver-related complications can be life-threatening, most of the time this inflammation is mild and does not constitute a major problem. Many children who acquire liver problems will experience nothing more than mild elevations of liver enzymes. Other children can develop scarring of the liver or the ducts. Other than discontinuing the use of medications that might be aggravating them, there really is no treatment for these conditions. Among drug-related causes of these problems are medications containing 5-aminosalicylic such as Azulfidine®.

Renal or kidney-related complications also occur. Strictly speaking, since they arise in conjunction with severe inflammatory conditions throughout the GI tract, some of these are not typical extraintestinal manifestations. In Crohn's disease, where inflammation in the right lower quadrant occurs, a blockage of the right ureter or right kidney may develop. This blockage generally responds to a more aggressive therapy. A small percentage of patients will develop kidney stones.

COMPLICATIONS IN GENERAL

Doctors cannot determine ahead of time which children with inflammatory bowel disease will go on to develop complications. Most of the time these complications tend to appear in those whose IBD-related problems have tended to be severe from the beginning. However, complications, most of which tend to manifest themselves later in life, can occur in any individual case at any time.

COMPLICATIONS WITH FISTULAS AND ABSCESSES

Fistulas are limited to Crohn's disease and are caused by the underlying disease process itself. At times Crohn's-related inflammation will break through the intestinal wall and make a fistula, an abnormal tract connecting to some other structure. The most common fistula occurs when a looped segment of the intestine connects with another looped area. Though a fistula may be difficult to locate, fistula development should be suspected when a child is not responding to therapy or is experiencing unusual symptoms. The best way to investigate for fistulas is with a barium X-ray, either via a small bowel series or, if the large intestine is suspected, a barium enema. Though less frequently than adults, children do at times acquire intestine-to-intestine fistulas. Young people are also known to develop fistulas to the urinary bladder or to the abdominal wall. Fistulas to the bladder can cause urinary infections or the sensation of passing air in the urine. A fistula that ends blindly or does not "burrow" into another organ can be considered an abscess, a collection of pus in a walled-off area. These tend to occur when the bacteria normally found in the intestine manage to occupy another cavity.

Perianal fistulas and abscesses are fairly common among those with patients with Crohn's disease, occurring in approximately 15% of cases. These conditions can often be treated successfully with sitz baths or soaking the perianal area in a warm bath, with or without added salts. When a perianal abscess develops, it will eventually point and drain to the skin, becoming a fistula. The latter respond very well to treatment with antibiotics or steroids, and 6-mercaptopurine seems to be very beneficial for chronic perianal fistulas. In a small number of children, fistulas can become very aggressive and disfiguring.

Fistulas and abscesses occurring in other parts of the intestinal tract can be refractory. Though generally initially responsive to antibiotics and steroids, they sometimes recur and eventually require intravenous therapy. Surgery often becomes necessary. Such surgery frequently entails the removal of the involved segment of bowel. These possible complications coupled with poor outcome after surgery are among the reasons that physicians are often inclined to provide some children with a trial of immunosuppressive drugs before considering surgery. Even if the child's response to medication is slow and discouraging, children and parents should be encouraged to exercise patience. Surgical therapy, the other option, may "cure" the problem temporarily, only to have the fistula return at a later date. Total bowel rest with parenteral nutrition is an effective form of therapy in some individuals, but abscesses or collections of pus in the abdomen need to be treated with antibiotics. Surgical drainage may also be necessary.

STRICTURES

Strictures are circumferential scarrings of the bowel that narrow it and restrict the passage of intestinal contents. In cases of possible stricture formation, a trial of medical therapy under the close supervision of a physician may determine whether or not a problem is a true stricture or simply an area of spasm related to inflammation. Stricture symptoms usually involve either vomiting or a sense of fullness after eating or drinking. At times, however, acute inflammation, which is not a stricture, produce similar symptoms.

The formation of strictures is more common decades after diagnosis and does not occur as readily in children as adults. Reasons for stricture development are unclear. While active inflammation tends to produce more of the acute symptoms of pain and diarrhea, chronic inflammation of the deeper intestinal layers seems to stimulate a scarring process.

Whenever a stricture does not respond to conventional medical therapy, surgical removal of the affected area is required. Problems occur when the physician discovers multiple strictures and does not want to resect large areas of intestine. Under these circumstances, some surgeons will use a technique called stricturoplasty. This is a surgical technique in which existing strictures are opened and resewn. In such instances, the luminal passage or interior of the intestine is widened and, ideally, the obstructive symptoms surgically excised. Unfortunately, stricture formation may recur following surgical therapy, even after the diseased region of the bowel is resected or surgically removed. For this reason, postoperative maintenance immunosuppressive therapy may be prescribed to prevent recurrence.

PERFORATION

A perforation of the bowel is a medical emergency. Fortunately, it is a rare event in children with inflammatory bowel disease. In Crohn's disease, a perforation is a slow process, generally associated with and preceded by fistula formation. The fistula may seal itself off, or it may burrow into another segment of the bowel, causing another fistula.

Perforation is an extremely rare complication of IBD in children. Perforations may, however, occur in children with Crohn's disease who are undergoing colonoscopy or enemas. If a potent form of medical treatment is carried out for a long period of time, especially in ulcerative colitis, the bowel wall becomes weakened and perforation may occur. Actual perforation requires surgical resection on an emergency basis. This is one of the reasons why specialists prefer to schedule an "elective" resection as soon as a severely weakened bowel wall is discovered.

CARCINOMA

Carcinoma is rare in children and adults with Crohn's disease. After a decade of disease, however, individuals with ulcerative colitis face increased risks of developing a carcinoma or cancer. For that reason, doctors typically schedule screening colonoscopies accompanied by multiple biopsies on a regular basis a decade after the onset of ulcerative colitis. Early detection of changes that suggest the development of cancer is the best way to prevent the occurrence and development of a malignancy. Carcinoma is mostly a concern in longstanding ulcerative colitis, though in recent years it has been found in some adults with severe colonic Crohn's. The initial data indicate that with each decade of ulcerative colitis, there is a 10% cumulative incidence of carcinoma. Regular surveillance is generally recommended. More recent data would seem to indicate that when surveillance colonoscopies are routinely performed, and when patients with more severe ulcerative colitis have colectomies, the overall risk of carcinoma is not as high as would be initially suggested. (The study referred to above was based on a retrospective analysis.) However, it is because some risk of carcinoma remains that those children with severe ulcerative colitis and borderline responses to medical therapy may ultimately be better off with surgery, essentially curing the illness, eliminating the side effects of the medications, and greatly reducing the risk of future malignancy.

CHAPTER 9

SURGERY

Except in instances of obstruction or for extraintestinal symptoms or other special complications, elective surgery is rarely performed in Crohn's disease because the symptoms tend to recur afterwards. In ulcerative colitis, however, surgery can cure the disease. Although many IBD patients view surgery as a failure of medical therapy, the surgeon is an important member of the medical team and should be involved with disease management, even when the need for surgery may not arise.

Surgical intervention is needed in ulcerative colitis when medical therapy is unable to control a specific acute problem, such as bleeding. The risk of developing colon cancer with ulcerative colitis may also become a factor in a decision to choose surgery. The form of therapy ultimately selected will result from each child and family member carefully weighing the potential risks and benefits. Opinions of pediatric gastroenterologists, pediatric surgeons, health care providers, nurse specialists, and nutritionists can prove invaluable in helping children and their families make these decisions.

During the last 20 years, the surgical management of ulcerative colitis has evolved. Operations that maintain anal function have increasingly become the standard of care. The need for a permanent ileostomy and an appliance worn on the abdomen to collect intestinal drainage in patients with ulcerative colitis is all but unheard of today.

The timing of surgery will depend on the initial presentation of the disease, responsiveness to treatment, and the level of the child's and family's acceptance of the need for surgical therapy. Three conditions lead to surgery in children with ulcerative colitis:

1. A surgical emergency, usually caused by a rapid dilation of the colon or perforation of the bowel or uncontrollable hemorrhage.
2. Disease that is not responsive to optimal medical management.
3. Disease that is debilitating and chronic, causing an unacceptable quality of life.

INDICATIONS FOR SURGERY

1. Surgical emergency
   A. Colonic perforation
   B. Uncontrolled colonic hemorrhage
2. Severe disease unresponsive to medical management
   A. Toxic megacolon
   B. Continued severe symptoms after 2 weeks of maximum support including IV steroids and cyclosporine
3. Unacceptable quality of life
   A. Recurrent or intractable colitis
   B. Growth failure
   C. Intractable extraintestinal manifestations
   D. Morbidity from long-term systemic steroids
   E. Risk for developing colonic cancer

Most of the time, surgical intervention is required for uncontrolled colonic bleeding or for a failure to achieve an initial remission in the patient, despite high doses of steroids and bowel rest. Of the conditions that lead to surgery because they are unresponsive to medical management, toxic megacolon is the most acute and, fortunately, the least common. Signs of toxic megacolon include high fever, a heightened white blood cell count, a large fluid requirement, and thrombocytopenia (an abnormal decrease in blood platelets). If perforation is imminent, surgery may be required within 48 to 72 hours of these initial symptoms. Any delay in recognizing and treating this condition may be truly life threatening.

The indications for surgery in cases of colonic hemorrhage or failure to achieve remission are fairly clear cut. However, decisions favoring surgery due to an unacceptable quality of life are necessarily made on much more subjective grounds. School attendance and participation in extracurricular activities, family satisfaction, and the child's tolerance of disease symptoms are all highly important factors in such a decision. So, too, are growth failure, delayed development of sexual maturity, intractable and painful extraintestinal manifestations, and the risk of morbidity from long-term steroid usage.

The decision to undergo surgery for chronic debilitating disease during the tumultuous teenage years should be made only after detailed discussions involving the patient, parents, surgeon, pediatric gastroenterologist, therapist, and nurse specialist. Those contemplating this choice should be encouraged to discuss the prospects of surgery with other young people who have undergone a similar operation.

The development of cancer is also a very real concern for patients with ulcerative colitis. While the risk is quite low during the first decade of the disease, it increases over time. The occurrence of carcinoma is more common among patients with pancolitis and chronic inflammation. People who develop ulcerative colitis as children must remain under close medical observation as they become adults. Mild or limited disease does not obviate the ultimate risk of colon cancer.

A CHILD WHO REQUIRED SURGICAL THERAPY

A 16-year old girl presented with a two-month history of intermittent bloody stools. One week before hospital admission, she developed diarrhea and fever. Sigmoidoscopy revealed severe diffuse active ulcerative colitis. Stool cultures, examination for ova and parasites, and a tuberculin skin test were obtained. The results were all negative. Three days before admission to the hospital she developed nausea, vomiting, and a poor appetite. At the time of admission, she was feverish with a mildly distended, tender abdomen. Her white blood cell count was elevated at $16,700/mm^3$ with a KUB that demonstrated an absence of colonic markings (natural sac-like pouches of the colon), but no significant increase in the size of the bowel. Intravenous (IV) antibiotics and high-dose steroids were started and food was withheld while she was provided with nutrition by vein. Despite these therapies, as well as a trial of prednisone and cyclosporine, more than 1 quart of bloody diarrhea per day persisted over the next week, requiring multiple blood transfusions. A barium upper gastrointestinal (GI) study was entirely normal and provided no evidence of Crohn's disease. At this time, a catheter was placed into a large vein in her chest so higher amounts of calories could be provided and her weight could be stabilized.

Discussions were started with the young girl and her family about the possibility of surgery. The surgeon who had been involved with her care and her pediatric gastroenterologist began to describe in greater detail how the operation was performed. As bleeding continued, both the girl and her family wanted to learn more about surgery. At the same time, they became more anxious. Questions came up about how an appliance would function, if she could go to school, what her friends would think, if she should take gym, and how it would feel not to have a colon. A therapist came to speak with the girl on a regular basis about her concerns and worries. A child who had previously undergone the operation and returned to school came to visit. The enterostomal nurse provided models demonstrating how her intestine would work and the proposed location of the appliance. The patient wore the appliance for a day to see how it felt.

By the end of the second week in the hospital, her weight was stable from the nutrition, but she felt terrible from all the medication. What was worse, she was still passing 10 bloody stools each day, getting up at night to go to the bathroom, and still having blood transfusions. She decided that she wanted to have surgery, and her therapist felt she was ready to make this decision.

An abdominal colectomy (removal of part or all of the colon), Brooke ileostomy (severing of the ileum and the creation of a permanent surgical opening in the abdomen through which feces can empty), and closure of the rectal stump was performed 19 days after admission. Six months later, she had an ileoanal pull-through with a diverting ileostomy. The ileostomy was closed at four months, and excellent continence has been achieved.

Surgical Management

A rapid evolution has occurred in the surgical management of ulcerative colitis. Currently several treatment alternatives are available to the patient and surgeon. Prior to 1950, colectomy, a removal of part or all of the colon, was seldom performed for ulcerative colitis. The very ill patient was previously subjected to some form of "venting" procedure, such as appendicostomy (irrigation of the cecum and colon), cecostomy (surgical creation of an artificial anus), or a double-barrel ileostomy through which various irrigants could be administered. The standard ileostomy of that era often resulted in serious inflammation of the exposed bowel wall, high stoma (artificial opening into the bowel) output, fluid and salt depletion, and severe and painful skin inflammation. Recognition of the need to perform a proctocolectomy (removal of all or part of the colon, rectum and anus) in order to provide a disease-free outcome, and improvements in the ileostomy techniques by surgeons, have constituted great advances. Recent efforts have focused on technical improvements and the achievement of fecal continence. Taken together, these surgical advances have greatly improved the patient's post-surgical quality of life.

The specific initial surgery is determined by the clinical condition of the child. In the acute setting when colonic resection is required for toxic megacolon, fulminant colitis hemorrhage, or perforation, the procedure may be limited to an abdominal colectomy, closure but not removal of the distal rectum, and a Brooke ileostomy, as in the case history described above. However, some surgeons can remove the diseased colon and create a rectal pouch in a single operation. When the acute episode is over, or if the surgery is not required by an emergency, several reconstructive procedures can be considered. The extent of the surgery is determined by the clinical situation and the expertise and experience of the surgeon. There is no one "best technique," and each surgeon develops and perfects individual methods. However, in 1996, the endorectal pull-through is the most favored operation.

SURGERY IN THE ACUTE SETTING

Colectomy and Brooke ileostomy are the operations of choice in the acute setting for ulcerative colitis, because they are associated with the lowest frequency of complications and can be accomplished most expeditiously in the acutely ill patient. Major drawbacks are the external stoma and a required appliance. Colectomy with a Brooke ileostomy is technically the simplest procedure for ulcerative colitis. In a recent review, revision was required in only 11% of patients. More than 90% of the adult patients who responded to a questionnaire stated they were

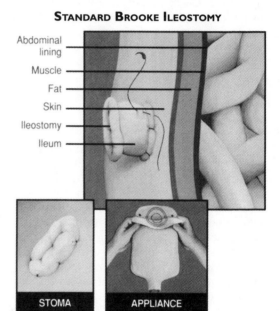

STANDARD BROOKE ILEOSTOMY

Abdominal lining
Muscle
Fat
Skin
Ileostomy
Ileum

STOMA

APPLIANCE

satisfied with their diets, were employed, and had few problems with the management of their stomas. About 75% of the responding patients experienced no restrictions in daily activities, and 95% expressed overall satisfaction with the surgery and ileostomy. The majority stated they would not consider a change in the type of ileostomy they had, despite negative responses to the considerable cost of stoma supplies. Other negative responses included peristomal skin irritations (around the edges of the surgical opening) during their postoperative course, while persistent unhealed perineal wounds (around the anal opening) occurred in about 33% of the patients. Perhaps the most telling aspect of these reports is that many patients aware of alternative procedures either desire or would consider a surgical alternative. Adolescents are particularly reluctant to accept a permanent ileostomy.

In ulcerative colitis, permanent ileostomy need not be considered. However, at the time of surgery, it may not be possible to know if the patient has ulcerative colitis or Crohn's colitis. When the colon is removed and the pathologist can inspect it carefully, features suggestive of Crohn's disease may be discovered. If this situation occurs, the risk of performing a pull-through is increased because Crohn's could flare up in the remaining small intestine. Most surgeons will not perform a pull-through operation if a diagnosis of Crohn's disease is established. However, there are unfortunate situations in which even the pathologist thinks the tissue looks like ulcerative colitis, only to discover that disease has returned in the remaining small intestine after surgery has been performed. If the patient has ulcerative colitis, the stoma or ileostomy can be replaced by an internal pouch that empties through the rectum. If the patient has Crohn's disease, the stoma that has been created will become a permanent ileostomy.

SURGERY IN THE ELECTIVE SETTING

The ileorectal anastomosis with preservation of the rectum has been a controversial alternative to proctocolectomy and the Brooke ileostomy and is not widely accepted. The major concerns raised about the ileorectal anastomosis have centered around leaving the involved rectal mucosa intact despite its known potential for malignant degeneration. Colorectal cancer has been reported in patients who are left with the rectal stump. The use of this procedure is generally reserved for special situations where a stoma or fecal incontinence would be difficult to manage. If ileorectal anastomosis is selected, close follow-up and periodic endoscopy are essential.

THE KOCK POUCH

The continent ileostomy or the Kock pouch was designed to free the patient of an ostomy device while still allowing drainage of a stoma on the abdominal wall. A reservoir is

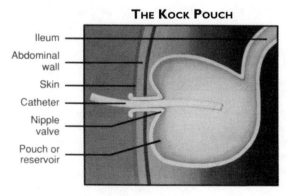

THE KOCK POUCH

Ileum
Abdominal wall
Skin
Catheter
Nipple valve
Pouch or reservoir

created from the terminal portion of the ileum, with the addition of a nipple valve that allows egress of pouch contents only when intubated by a specially constructed ileostomy catheter.

The major advantage of this method consists of the avoidance of an external ostomy device. Major disadvantages are threefold. First, the Kock pouch requires intubation by the patient on a regular schedule, a demand often difficult for the teenage patient to manage. Second, it requires manipulation of the stoma, which is often as disagreeable to the child as dealing with the ostomy device. Finally, even in the best of hands, the procedure has been plagued by the need for surgical revision. For these reasons, the Kock pouch has not been used significantly in the pediatric population.

THE ILEOANAL PULL-THROUGH

The ileoanal pull-through (also called the ileal pouch-anal anastomosis) is another surgical alternative. Since the technical details of the procedure have been established and favorable results have been reported, it has gained in favor. Key technical factors for successful ileoanal pull-through include the creation of some reservoir capacity. Placement of the pouch within the pelvis below the peritoneal floor results in improved emptying. Removal of the rectal mucosa in ulcerative colitis is difficult because the inflamed friable (easily broken) mucosa makes this a very lengthy and tedious procedure. A rectal muscular cuff of 5 to 6 cm has proved adequate for continence.

Establishing continence can be complex. Without the colon to reabsorb water, the stool will be liquid in contrast with the normal consistency of stool. Studies have shown that ileal capacity, compliance, and complete emptying correlate very well with good functional outcome. Reservoir capacity is achieved through either construction of a pouch or dilation of the ileum. Finally, the sphincters and other muscles involved with continence must be preserved and not damaged during surgery. Following surgery and the creation of a reservoir, the creation of a stoma to divert the stream of stool away from the newly made pouch may be necessary. This temporary ileostomy remains in place until the pouch heals. During this time, some surgeons and pediatric gastroenterologists will recommend exercises to strengthen the muscles and train the pouch to hold liquid. Once the diverting ileostomy is removed, permitting the stool to flow into the pouch, the muscles around the anal canal must be strong enough to hold back the stool or the patient will be incontinent and leak stool. As the patient learns to control these muscles, the reservoir gets larger, the muscles become stronger, and episodes of leakage become less frequent. If a patient continues to have difficulties, underlying problems such as inflammation in the pouch

ILLUSTRATION OF ILEOANAL PULL-THROUGH

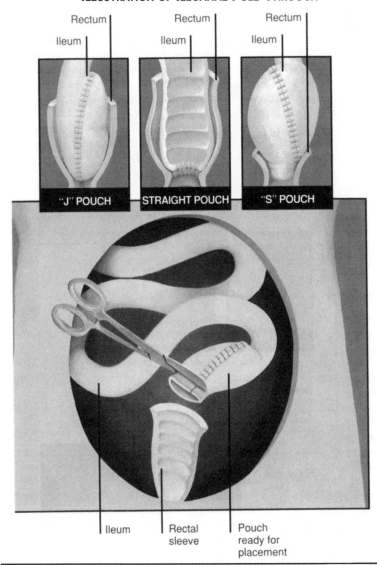

Rectum | Rectum | Rectum
Ileum | Ileum | Ileum

"J" POUCH   STRAIGHT POUCH   "S" POUCH

Ileum   Rectal sleeve   Pouch ready for placement

could be responsible. Biofeedback techniques can be helpful in training these muscles and improving function.

The most important concerns for patients after surgery center
around the adequacy of fecal continence. Stool frequency is generally

of secondary importance. The success of the procedure has varied, but several centers have reported good results. Pediatric populations have reported no major difficulties with daytime leakage and a 3 to 13% occurrence of nocturnal leakage requiring the use of a pad. In one report, only 3 of 65 patients required subsequent ileostomy and were considered poor results, while only 2 patients had persistent moderate nocturnal soiling lasting more than 6 months following surgery. Some surgeons have utilized the straight ileoanal anastomosis without a pouch and preserved the distal 1 cm of rectal mucosa. Patients so treated also have been continent during the daytime and only rarely incontinent at night. However, as has been mentioned, preservation of rectal mucosa creates potential risks of cancer later in life. Stool frequency ranges from 2 to 20 stools per day shortly after surgery.

Some patients have required psyllium hydrophilic mucilloid (Metamucil®), diphenoxylate-atropine (Lomotil®), and loperamide (Imodium®) to decrease the frequency of bowel movements after surgery. Because of postoperative enlargement and accommodation of the pouch, this frequency usually decreases to an average of six movements per day after a year.

OPERATIONS FOR CROHN'S DISEASE: BOWEL RESECTION

If an area of the intestine is narrowed (usually, but not always, the small intestine) and causes chronic abdominal pain or bowel obstruction, or if there is a connection from one part of the bowel to another (a fistula), a consideration of surgical removal may be discussed with the patient and family. Sometimes medical therapy can reduce the inflammation and increase the opening so digesting food does not block the bowel. Special diets of low residue foods, or liquid nutritional supplements can also be tried. However, if these therapies are unsuccessful, removal of the narrowed region may be necessary. The concern about removing a portion of the bowel is that Crohn's disease can recur in a previously healthy segment of the bowel. If the bowel continues to be removed, however, there may come a time when there is no longer enough remaining bowel to absorb food, resulting in an interference with normal growth and physical maturation. For this reason, careful consideration of medical options should be studied prior to a decision to proceed with surgical resection for strictures and fistulas.

STRICTUROPLASTY

When multiple areas of narrowing are present or there exists a single restricted area of the bowel, it may be possible to widen the affected portion of bowel. This operation is performed by cutting the outside of the narrowed segment and then resewing it perpendicular to the original incision. This shortens the segment, but enlarges the lumen of the bowel through which the digesting food flows. Decisions about this procedure will depend on the location of the disease, the history of previous surgery, the risk of complications such as fistulas (connections between loops of bowel), and the length of the narrowing. This type of operation has had limited use in children.

SUMMARY

Surgical emergency, disease unresponsive to medical management, and an unacceptable quality of life are the general indications for surgery in patients with ulcerative colitis. Currently, several surgical alternatives are available to the child who may elect surgery. Each procedure has limitations. Modification of the techniques will continue as additional experience is gained. A full discussion of each surgical possibility with the patient and family is essential to making the best choice and preparing the child and family for possible complications. When an emergency colectomy is required, the rectum should be retained to allow for the future option of choosing an ileoanal pull-through. Involvement of nurse specialists, mental health professionals, nutritionists, and supportive parents is critical when it comes to providing information to the patient and child about surgical options. Surgery in children with Crohn's disease is usually undertaken only when medical therapy has failed to resolve bowel obstructions or extraintestinal complications such as fistulas or abscesses.

CHAPTER 10

THE ROLE OF DIET

Even before the onset of gastrointestinal symptoms, young people with inflammatory bowel disease may not have been growing as well as healthy children. In addition, owing to chronic diarrhea or fevers, young patients are likely to have increased food requirements. Finally, children with IBD may be required to take medications that interfere with normal appetites. For these reasons it is highly important that these children be provided with a well-balanced diet. Unless an intestinal obstruction or other problem is present, a child's food intake should not be restricted. In most instances, at least, "bowel rest" has no place in the contemporary treatment of mild to moderate IBD.

AN APPROPRIATE DIET

An appropriate diet should be drawn from all food groups. Meat, fish, poultry, and dairy products, if tolerated, are sources of protein; bread, cereal, starches, fruits, and vegetables are sources of carbohydrates; margarine and oils are sources of fat. Your physician and a registered dietitian can help with meal planning.

FLUID INTAKE

A child whose condition is characterized by chronic diarrhea runs the risk of dehydration, a condition characterized by salt loss and a feeling of weakness. If fluid intake does not keep up with a child's diarrhea, kidney function may be affected. For this reason, children with IBD should consume ample fluids, especially in warm weather when skin losses of salt and water may be high. Patients with Crohn's disease have an increased incidence of kidney stones, partly attributable to dehydration. Thankfully, kidney stones are unusual in young people.

SPECIFIC DIET THERAPY

Even under ordinary circumstances, the nutritional needs of children and adolescents are known to exceed those of fully grown adults. The nutritional requirements of children with inflammatory bowel disease are greater still and, in fact, are estimated to be about 1.5 times the ordinary recommended daily allowances (RDA). The recommended daily allowance can be thought of as the nutrition necessary to meet the known needs of a healthy individual. For the child with IBD, this breaks down to an average daily intake of approximately 35 calories per pound of body weight per day. Daily intake of protein should be about 1 to 1.5 grams per pound.

LACTOSE

Many people believe that lactose, the sugar present in milk or dairy products, should be avoided by those with IBD. In some cases, this is true. However, studies have shown that lactose intolerance, which results in abdominal pain, diarrhea, or flatulence, is no more common among IBD patients than among the general population. For this reason, dairy products should be restricted only for children known to suffer from lactose intolerance. Even so, it is also true (and should count for something) that some lactose-intolerant people, especially children and teenagers, think an occasional sundae or some other highly desirable food is worth a certain amount of subsequent discomfort.

FIBER

Fiber may be helpful to some children with inflammatory bowel disease and detrimental to others. Certain foods such as bran cereal, legumes, dried fruit, apples, and pears may contain as much as 3–4 grams of dietary fiber per serving. Whenever Crohn's disease is accompanied by a narrowing of the bowel, children may need to avoid fiber, especially nuts and popcorn. However, there is no reason for your child to avoid fiber-containing foods. unless the child's physician has a specific reason for denying them.

NUTRITIONAL SUPPLEMENTS

Sometimes, simply urging a child to eat can result in an improved intake of nutrients. If, however, children with IBD cannot eat enough to sustain or gain desirable weight, or if they are deficient in vitamins and essential minerals, specific nutritional supplementation may be required (see page 82). Dietary supplementation may consist of highly caloric

SPECIFIC NUTRIENTS

NUTRIENT	REASON FOR SUPPLEMENTATION
Calcium	Treatment with steroids
	Malabsorption
Fat Soluble Vitamins	
Vitamin A, D, E, K	Malabsorption
Folate	Sulfa-containing medications
Iron	Anemia, blood loss
Zinc	Diarrhea
Multivitamins	
with minerals	Increased requirements
Magnesium	Malabsorption

SUPER CALORIE DRINKS
(CALORIE/PROTEIN AMOUNTS GIVEN FOR 1-CUP SERVINGS)

Note: Some of these drinks are easily prepared in a blender. All should be consumed immediately after preparation or immediately refrigerated for later consumption. After three days, unconsumed drinks should be discarded.

High Protein Milk
1 cup whole milk
4 tablespoons dry milk powder
= 1 serving, 210 calories, 14 gm protein

High Protein Milkshake 1
1 cup High Protein milk
1 cup ice cream
½ teaspoon vanilla
= 2 servings, 298 calories, 10 gm protein

High Protein Milkshake 2
¾ High Protein Milk
1 cup ice cream
¼ Half and Half
2 tablespoons chocolate syrup
= 2 servings, 345 calories, 9 gm protein

Sherbet Shake
1½ cups sherbet
¼ cup whole milk
4 tablespoons dry milk
= 2 servings, 245 calories, 6 gm protein

Juice Shake
¾ cup pineapple or any juice
1½ cups ice cream
3 tablespoons dry milk powder
= 2 servings, 353 calories, 7 gm protein

Yogurt Milkshake
8 ounces fruited yogurt
1 package vanilla instant breakfast mix
1 cup High Protein milk
= 2 servings, 300 calories, 16 gm protein

Banana Milkshake
1½ bananas
1½ cups whole milk
3 drops vanilla
¼ cup Half and Half
3 tablespoons dry milk powder
= 2 servings, 270 calories, 11 gm protein

Fruit Shake
1 cup vanilla commercial liquid nutritional supplement
1 large banana or other fruit
= 1 serving, 336 calories, 1 gm of protein

Milkshake
8 ounces commercial liquid nutritional supplement
1 cup ice cream
3 tablespoons chocolate syrup
= 1½ servings, 430 calories, 14 gm protein

Polycose Kool-aid
1 package Kool-aid
1 cup Polycose powder
= 2 quarts, 240 calories

Polycose Juice
1 cup clear juice (apple, cranberry, grape)
2 tablespoons Polycose powder
= 1 serving, 170 calories

Homemade Instant Breakfast
1 cup High Protein milk
2 tablespoons chocolate syrup
= 1 serving, 285 calories, 15 gm protein

U. S. Department of Agriculture, U. S. Department of Health and Human Services. *Nutrition and Your Health, Dietary Guidelines for Americans*, Lloyd-Still JD (ed): *Textbook of Cystic Fibrosis*, Boston: John Wright, 1983.

drinks (see page 82–83), foods high in protein (see page 85), foods containing high amounts of fat (see page 85), or carbohydrates (see page 86). For suggestions of high-calorie snacks, see pages 86 and 87. If the doctor or nutritionist feels it is necessary, a specific nutritional supplement can be prescribed on a daily basis. Pages 87 and 88 provide an example of a high-calorie protein meal plan.

Very often, a child's IBD may make consuming food or drink supplements difficult or impossible. For one thing, supplementation may detract from what the child would eat at ordinary meals. For another, supplements may cause gastrointestinal symptoms such as pain, diarrhea, or vomiting. Finally, although several flavors are available, taste fatigue is a common problem with day-to-day intake of the same supplement. If necessary, overnight tube feedings can also be used to supply nutrients.

ENTERAL TUBE FEEDING

Either because they interfere with a child's eating regular meals or induce vomiting, diarrhea, or pain, extra supplements by mouth do not always succeed in inducing desirable growth in children who lack an appetite. In such instances, infusing certain formulas directly into the gastrointestinal tract via tube can be helpful. The most common method for doing this is via nasogastric feeding.

In nasogastric tube feeding, the tube goes through the nose, through the esophagus, and into the stomach. There are two methods of nasogastric tube feeding. The nocturnal tube is placed each night and removed each morning. Alternatively, the indwelling tube is placed by a doctor or nurse and remains in place as long as necessary. Many doctors will teach a young adult or a family member to pass the tube by themselves.

Nasogastric feeding does not require surgery and is often effective for short-term use. Nocturnal usage enables the patient to

NASOGASTRIC TUBE FEEDING

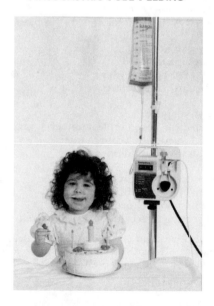

CALORIE-PACKING FOODS

FOOD	CALORIES PER TBSP.	USE IN or ON:
PROTEINS:		
Peanut butter	94	Bread, crackers, toast, raw fruit, vegetables, milkshake
Cheese	50	Vegetables, casseroles, meats, sandwiches, dips, soups, salads
Dry milk powder	25	Whole milk, mashed potatoes, scrambled eggs, ground beef, casseroles, pudding, yogurt, creamed soup, milkshakes
Egg yolks	60	Meatloaf, baked goods, sandwich spreads, salads

U. S. Department of Agriculture, U. S. Department of Health and Human Services. *Nutrition and Your Health, Dietary Guidelines for Americans,* Lloyd-Still JD (ed): *Textbook of Cystic Fibrosis,* Boston: John Wright, 1983.

CALORIE-PACKING FATS

FOOD	CALORIES PER TBSP.	USE IN or ON:
*Oil	25	Baby foods, infant formulas, hot cereal, soups, vegetables,
(MCT oil)	115	casseroles
Margarine	100	Hot cereal, vegetables, soups, sandwiches, casseroles, mashed potatoes, breads
Sour cream	26	Vegetables, salads, casseroles, dips
Cream cheese	50	Toast, bagel, sandwiches, scrambled eggs, raw vegetables
Mayonnaise	100	Salads, sandwiches, deviled eggs, vegetables
Chopped nuts	50	Pudding, ice cream, salads, casseroles, cereal, baked goods, desserts
Gravy	26	Meats, mashed potatoes, pasta casseroles, vegetables
Cream	60	Cereal, hot chocolate, milk, casseroles, goods, pudding, jello

*   *No more than 2 tablespoons oil per day if less than 2 years of age. No more than 3 tablespoons oil per day if 3 years or older.*

U. S. Department of Agriculture, U. S. Department of Health and Human Services. *Nutrition and Your Health, Dietary Guidelines for Americans,* Lloyd-Still JD (ed): *Textbook of Cystic Fibrosis,* Boston: John Wright, 1983.

CALORIE-PACKING CARBOHYDRATES

FOOD	CALORIES PER TBSP.	USE IN or ON:
Karo Syrup/Honey*	60	Cereal, beverages, fruit milkshakes
Jam, jelly, syrup	52	Bread, toast, baked goods, ice cream
Chocolate syrup	45	Ice cream, beverages, cereal
Polycose/Moducal	23-30	Beverages, spaghetti sauce, gravy, yogurt, pudding

* Not recommended for infants less than 1 year old.

U. S. Department of Agriculture, U. S. Department of Health and Human Services. *Nutrition and Your Health, Dietary Guidelines for Americans*, Lloyd-Still JD (ed): *Textbook of Cystic Fibrosis*, Boston: John Wright, 1983.

HIGH CALORIE SNACKS

250 Calories

Corn muffin and jam	245
Chocolate malt	245
Baked custard	235
1 slice devil's food cake	250
1 cup chocolate pudding	250

500 Calories

1 cup dry cereal	160
1 banana	90
1 cup whole milk	160
1 slice toast	70
1 teaspoon butter	90
TOTAL	**570**

6 Graham crackers	100
2 tablespoons peanut butter	190
½ cup dried fruit	200
TOTAL	**490**

8 saltine crackers	100
1 ounce cheese	75
1 cup ice cream	290
TOTAL	**465**

8 ounces yogurt	240
4 tablespoons raisins	105
2 tablespoons wheat germ	50
¼ cup walnuts	200
TOTAL	**595**

750 plus calories

Ice cream sundae

2 scoops ice cream	270
4 tablespoons of chocolate syrup	250
3 tablespoons whipped cream	90
¼ cup walnuts	200
TOTAL	**810**

Roast beef sandwich

2 slices bread	140
4 ounces roast beef	300
2 teaspoons catsup	30
2 teaspoons mayonnaise	90
6 chocolate chip cookies	200
TOTAL	**760**

2 slices pizza	290
with extra cheese	200
8 ounces cola	90
1 cup chocolate pudding	285
TOTAL	**875**

U. S. Department of Agriculture, U. S. Department of Health and Human Services. *Nutrition and Your Health, Dietary Guidelines for Americans,* Lloyd-Still JD (ed): *Textbook of Cystic Fibrosis,* Boston: John Wright, 1983.

SAMPLE HIGH-CALORIE PROTEIN MEAL PLAN

BREAKFAST	**Calories**
1 cup orange juice	80
1 cup cereal with ½ cup whole milk	150
1 tablespoon raisins	30
2 slices bread	140
2 teaspoons jam	60
2 teaspoons margarine	90
1 banana	90
	Total: 720

(Continued on next page)

LUNCH	Calories
1 cup whole milk	160
2 slices bread	140
3 ounces turkey	165
2 teaspoons mayonnaise	90
15 potato chips	250
	Total: 1075

DINNER	
1 cup whole milk	160
5 -ounce steak	275
1 baked potato	70
1 tablespoon sour cream	70
½ cup broccoli with margarine	120
¾ cup strawberries	40
1 slice chocolate cake	235
	Total: 900

TOTAL FOR 3 MEALS: 2,695

---

receive nutrition at night and then, after removing the tube, eat, attend school, and carry on a normal life. However, nasogastric feeding can induce occasional vomiting. In addition, the patient can experience some irritation from passing the tube each night. Finally, a delay in eating may occur in young children. Of particular importance to many adolescents is the fact that because it is left in place, the indwelling tube (which is not removed), can be seen on the face and is likely to elicit comments from friends and strangers.

GASTROSTOMY TUBE FEEDING

When conditions are such that prolonged enteral feedings may be necessary, gastrostomy tube feedings may be preferable to nasogastric feedings. This approach calls for the insertion of tubes directly into the stomach. Two methods are commonly employed to place gastrostomy tubes directly into the stomach. The first method is known as percutaneous endoscopic gastrostomy (PEG). It can be accomplished endoscopically and does not require an abdominal incision. The second method, surgical gastrostomy, requires a minor incision.

Gastrostomy feedings provide greater mobility than nasogastric feedings. Additionally, patients are spared the irritation of passing the tube each night. Gastrostomy feedings also provide privacy. The small flat tubes on the stomach, not easily seen even through a bathing suit, mean that no tube will be visible on the face. The tubes can be placed while the patient is sedated or provided with general anesthesia. PEG feedings involve less pain than the surgically placed G-Tube, so patients can begin receiving nutrition within 24 hours. The surgically placed G-Tube has few advantages over the PEG-approach. Since gastrostomy feeding is invasive and tube placement sometimes requires anesthesia, usage brings a small risk of infection and minor complications. Some gastroenterologists have expressed concerns that the gastrostomy site might not close after the tube is removed. It is also possible that a Crohn's patient may develop an inflammation at the tube site.

JEJUNAL TUBE FEEDING

Another form of tube feeding, nasojejunal tubes, can sometimes alleviate problems of vomiting. Jejunal tubes are positioned in the small bowel. With the aid of medication, a nasojejunal tube is inserted in the nose, passed through the stomach and placed in the small bowel. It can be introduced by a radiologist using fluoroscopy or placed during an endoscopy. A feeding jejunostomy is a tube directed to the small bowel via the abdominal wall. Since these tubes bypass the stomach, there is virtually no vomiting. With the nasojejunal tube, aspiration, vomiting, and reflux are unlikely. In fact, nutrition can be introduced even if vomiting is present. The stomach can be decompressed with suction while nutrients are delivered to the small bowel. With the feeding jejunostomy, no tube is visible on the face. Both types of jejunal tubes must be placed by medical personnel. It sometimes happens that the tube becomes dislodged and must be repositioned, again by medical personnel. At best, these tubes are useful only in the hospital and are impractical for long-term use.

PARENTERAL NUTRITION

Parenteral nutrition, abbreviated to PN or sometimes total parenteral nutrition (TPN), consists of the delivery of nutrients directly into the blood. In most cases, nutrients are provided through an IV needle inserted in a peripheral vein. Sometimes nutrition is delivered through a major blood vessel by inserting a catheter through a vein in the neck and tunneling it down into a large blood vessel in the chest. Parenteral nutrition should only be used if oral supplements and enteral feedings are not tolerated or indicated. For the most part, PN serves as an adjunct to overall treatment and is impractical or dangerous to continue for long periods of time. While this approach, when warranted, can be highly beneficial, parenteral nutrition requires that a responsible individual pay very careful attention, both to the composition of the nutrient fluids and the insertion technique used to deliver them into the body. Since infections and other complications do occur in these feedings, PN is generally used for very specific indications. Doctors might consider PN when a patient is suffering from bowel obstruction, or when a patient is awaiting surgery for strictures or fistulas, or to provide time for medications and other treatments to begin reducing severe inflammation.

CHAPTER 11

TREATING SLOW GROWTH THROUGH NUTRITION

Slow growth in children has already been discussed as one of the symptoms of Crohn's disease and ulcerative colitis. Here we are concerned with its medical treatment. Slow growth can usually be treated effectively, even in instances where the reasons for its occurrence are less than fully understood.

Although puberty may be delayed by several years owing to the onset of inflammatory bowel disease, most teenagers with IBD do eventually reach maturity and function normally. Some individuals continue to gain height and weight into their twenties, after the onset of puberty and long after their peers have stopped growing. Many reach their "normal" height in this way.

Growth impairment is more common in Crohn's disease than in ulcerative colitis. It has been estimated that between 35 and 55% of children with Crohn's disease experience growth impairment; this compares with an incidence of between 5 and 10% growth impairment in patients with ulcerative colitis. Some children with IBD have tried growth hormone replacement as part of experimental protocols, but there has been no widespread conclusion about the effectiveness of growth hormone in inducing growth. In any case, hormonal deficiency does not appear with any consistency among IBD patients.

Some researchers have postulated that growth failure may be attributable to an excessive need for calories caused by chronic inflammation. Proponents of this view believe that calories sufficient for a normal individual are inadequate for a patient with inflammatory bowel disease. Others argue to the contrary, that growth failure in children with IBD results from maldigestion, a loss of, or an acquired inability to absorb and metabolize food already eaten. Both views have merit and, in fact, each of these factors may contribute to growth retardation.

MALNUTRITION

Inadequate Caloric Intake

Increased Losses

Malabsorption

Increased Requirements

The most common cause for growth failure, however, seems to be chronic undernutrition. Even when encouraged to eat more, many children with inflammatory bowel disease commonly feel full and lack hunger. Eating large meals can produce significant pain or discomfort, and children and adolescents who find this to be true seem to condition themselves to consume less and so reduce the discomfort that follows eating. Not surprisingly, in many instances, habits of reduced food intake often precede an IBD diagnosis by many years.

It is also true that since the medical goal in treating slow-growing children with IBD is to increase their height and weight and bring about physical maturation, a discussion of growth failure in terms of body weight alone could easily be misleading. In this regard, it has been documented that, in a child suffering from slow growth, weight gain must be sustained for several months before the child begins to grow taller and acquire characteristics of physical maturity. Disappointingly, while daily steroid treatments of children often increase the appetite, reduce inflammatory symptoms, make eating more pleasurable and eventually induce weight gain, increases in height and physical maturation often fail to occur. The appetite stimulation associated with steroids can be beneficial to children with poor appetites. However, it remains a matter of some frustration that steroids result in a gain of weight in the form of fat, rather than the increased lean body mass and muscle which are associated with the onset of physical maturity.

Delayed emptying of the stomach, documented in some children with Crohn's disease, is known to cause a sensation of being full. Malnutrition may also be exacerbated by bleeding and mucosal damage. The child may be experiencing losses in both protein and fat, as well as specific micronutrients such as iron, zinc, calcium, and magnesium. Contrary to some views, there does not seem to be a widespread need for an increased energy intake in many of these patients. Research indicates that the metabolic rates of children with IBD do not differ significantly from those demonstrated by controls. However, because they have a need to compensate for nutrient losses and make up for a failure in growth, children with inflammatory bowel disease have increased nutritional requirements. When adequate medical treatment relieves painful intestinal symptoms, IBD children eat better and resume growing.

Any deviation from a child's prior growth curve should be cause for concern. Height velocity, which is essentially the change in height over a given period, is the most precise method of detecting changes in growth patterns. Determinations of bone age by x-rays of the wrist can also be helpful in detecting growth failure and predicting future growth, as well as in measuring the success of recent therapy. Dual-energy x-ray absorptiometry (DEXA), is sometimes used to determine how well a patient's bones are mineralized. DEXA can also tell if an increase in weight consists of fat or muscle. Tanner staging, a method of assessing sexual maturation based on an examination of the genitalia and the distribution of body hair, can be of value with adolescents.

STAGES OF SEXUAL MATURITY IN GIRLS

Stage 1   Preadolescent pubic hair
Preadolescent breasts

Stage 2   Sparse pubic hair; lightly
pigmented, straight, medial
border of labia

Breast and papilla elevated as
small mound; areolar diameter
increase

Stage 3   Pubic hair darker; beginning to
curl, increased amount

Breast and areola enlarged, no
contour separation

Stage 4   Pubic hair coarse, curly,
abundant but amount less than
in adult

Areola and papilla form
secondary mound

Stage 5   Adult feminine triangle of pubic
hair, spread to medial surface of thighs

Mature breasts; nipple projects,
areola part of general breast
contour

STAGES OF SEXUAL MATURITY IN BOYS

Stage 1   No pubic hair
Preadolescent penis
Preadolescent testes

Stage 2   Scanty, long, slightly pigmented pubic hair
Slight enlargement of penis
Testes have enlarged scrotum with altered pink texture

Stage 3   Small amount of pubic hair which is darker and starts to curl
Longer penis
Larger testes

Stage 4   Pubic hair resembles adult type, but less in quantity; coarse, curly
Larger penis; glans and breadth increase in size
Larger testes, scrotum dark

Stage 5   Adult distribution of pubic hair, spread to medial surface of thighs
Adult penis
Adult testes

NUTRITIONAL FACTORS AS POTENTIAL ETIOLOGY FOR PEDIATRIC IBD

Many different theories have been advanced in an effort to answer questions about food and determine the role of nutrition in IBD. While there is no evidence that a poor diet causes IBD, the typical western diet is more commonly associated with IBD than African or Asian diets. In addition, immunological reactions to various foods have been studied in an effort to determine if some foods stimulate the overproduction of certain white blood cells and antibodies. Further investigations of this sort will have to be undertaken, however, before we can say with confidence that we know much about the role of foods and allergies in the development of IBD.

NUTRITIONAL DEFICIENCIES IN INFLAMMATORY BOWEL DISEASE

The most common nutritional deficiencies in children with inflammatory bowel disease consist of calories and protein rather than micronutrients. Insofar as they do occur, however, micronutrient deficiencies are more common among those with Crohn's disease. Folic acid, for example, can be deficient in patients with Crohn's disease, perhaps owing to an insufficient intake in a patient's diet. This folic acid insufficiency in children may or may not be accompanied by a diminished ability to absorb this vital nutrient. Folic acid deficiency is also known to be associated with the medication sulfasalazine, which interferes directly with the absorption of the nutrient. Comparable deficiencies of water soluble vitamins such as B-6, riboflavin, niacin, and vitamin C, are usually attributable to a lack of intake. However, vitamin B-12 deficiencies are commonly associated with ileal disease. This is especially so in instances of surgical resection (partial removal) of the bowel, as well as in cases characterized by bacterial overgrowth. Such deficiencies can occur in as many as 40% of children with Crohn's disease. A deficiency of fat-soluble vitamins (D, E, A, and K) is less common, and where present, usually occurs as a result of generalized fat malabsorption. A deficiency of calcium may also occur because of malabsorption. This deficiency is manifested by poor bone mineralization, a condition made worse by treatment with corticosteroids. A lack of iron is the most common deficiency. Unfortunately, because of ongoing intestinal losses and the irritating properties of iron preparations, an iron deficiency may prove difficult to treat in children.

A generalized deficiency in calories is frequently reflected in routine measurements, including height, weight, and skinfold thickness. Again, the major cause of growth failure appears to be a form of undernutrition, possibly but not necessarily attributable to disease activity or the use of corticosteroids.

The major thrust of nutritional therapy is to supply extra calories. At times, up to 150% of predicted caloric requirements are necessary to produce weight gain and reverse growth failure in a child with IBD. Efforts should always be made to provide these needed calories in the form of food. However, due to the nature of these illnesses and the reluctance of some children to eat foods which might make them uncomfortable, this strategy is not always successful. Nocturnal nasogastric feedings can be useful because they provide caloric intake at a time when the child would not ordinarily be receiving nutrition.

THE USE OF ELEMENTAL DIETS AS PRIMARY TREATMENT FOR IBD

The benefit of bowel rest and parenteral nutrition in IBD, ordinarily thought to be useful primarily in the treatment of ulcerative colitis, is not as clear for patients with Crohn's disease. Elemental formulas, specially constituted liquid meals without residue which contain all necessary nutrients, can be taken orally or via nasogastric tube. These feedings have been shown to increase weight and decrease disease activity as effectively as corticosteroid treatment. Many patients experiencing a flare up of Crohn's disease have been found to respond to an elemental diet and remain in remission after six months; however, recent analysis of well controlled studies has shown that corticosteroids were more effective overall than enteral nutrition and found no advantage to the use of elemental diets.

Adolescents, of course, are resistant to dietary restrictions and are understandably reluctant to drink unpalatable formulas. Therefore, while elemental diet treatments can be used to gain temporary remissions of symptoms without the use of corticosteroids, the long-term value and usefulness of these nutritional supplements remains unknown. For children unable to tolerate any food, however, total feeding by vein remains an option. Fortunately, for families with medical expenses, many states have laws requiring insurance carriers to pay for these nutritional supplements, just as they would be required to pay for other medications.

OVERALL DIETARY RECOMMENDATIONS

Other dietary recommendations can be quite subjective. Specific, restrictive diets aimed at eliminating certain foods from patient diets are regarded as monotonous by adolescents. This fact at least partly explains why these diets have not proven to be effective over a long period of time. As a general matter, decisions about what to eat and what to avoid eating should be made on an individual basis. Variable responses indicate that fiber and dairy products can be tolerated or even beneficial to some patients, while possibly deleterious to others. Lactose intolerance has been shown to be as widespread in the general population as it is among IBD patients. Moreover, since milk products can be valuable sources of calcium, protein, and calories, dairy products should be eliminated only from the diets of the demonstrably lactose intolerant. Vitamin and mineral supplements should be provided in conjunction with these feedings, both to maintain ordinary requirements and to compensate for any losses. However, specific supplements have not been scientifically shown to be effective in the management of slow growth unless deficiencies occur. Fish oil is a possible exception. Interestingly, fish oil seems to decrease the neutrophil production of the inflammatory mediator leukotriene. Some small studies have shown that the addition of 3 to 4 gms of fish oil to the diets of adults with IBD have produced clinical improvements in inflammation.

Maintaining adequate nutrition is crucial to the treatment of any chronic pediatric disease, especially diseases as closely linked to growth impairment as Crohn's disease and ulcerative colitis. When slow growth symptoms are persistent and extreme, the use of supplements that can be swallowed or taken via nasogastric feedings should be considered. Reinstating healthy appetites and stimulating appropriate physical growth and maturation are important.

PART III

LIVING WITH INFLAMMATORY BOWEL DISEASE

CHAPTER 12

REASSURING YOUR CHILD

Parents, older brothers and sisters, friends and school personnel should be helped to understand that young people with inflammatory bowel disease often resist being treated differently from their peers. Respect is important to a sense of personal well being, and in fact, there is no evidence to suggest that young people cope less well with Crohn's disease and ulcerative colitis than adults.

Unfortunately, it happens that some healthy young people are insensitive or lack the social skills necessary to help another person get through embarrassing moments. Thoughtlessness rather than cruelty is probably responsible for most of the embarrassing moments that adolescents inflict on one another. At times, children with inflammatory bowel disease faced with potentially humiliating situations withdraw from social interaction. The reasons for this are understandable: when social interaction carries a high potential for embarrassment, a child learns to be wary, sometimes choosing to remain isolated rather than risk the consequences of social thoughtlessness or deliberate cruelty.

When their diseases are active, young people with IBD may be reluctant to contact school officials and obtain special bathroom privileges or modified gym activities. In school environments where teachers and adults challenge any threatened disruption of classroom routine, it is not difficult to understand why a child may fear asking for permission to use the bathroom. Is it really any wonder that many young people with IBD are so strongly protective of their privacy?

Children with IBD very much need a safe and loving home environment and families who do all they can to provide comfort and protection. Loved and secure at home and among friends, children with IBD will be better equipped to deal with the problems they encounter as a result of having a chronic illness and feeling "different."

Occasional bouts of anger, anxiety, or depression are normal. However, parents should remain alert for signs of steady and persistent depression or anger. When a child's moods remain bleak and emotions are running high, professional attention from a social worker, psychologist, or psychiatrist can be very helpful.

Even among considerate and sympathetic friends, inflammatory bowel disease patients may be reluctant to discuss corticosteroids and other medications likely to create obvious changes in physical appearance. Although young people often avoid openly discussing IBD, even with close friends, they should be advised that such reticence is not always in their best interest. Familiarity with the CCFA's brochures for children, parents, and teachers may make discussing these issues easier for IBD patients. Through support groups, teenage patients of the same age and sex can reach out and find meaningful human contact. Parents, of course, should do what they can, short of nagging and pushiness, to encourage their children to seek out and nurture such relationships.

Young people often find it very difficult to discuss inflammatory bowel disease with health care providers. When interviewers ask about stool frequency, the presence of blood, or flatulence, adolescents are likely to regard

---

REACHING OUT

"Ulcerative colitis and Crohn's disease are bathroom diseases and no one wants to talk about a bathroom disease. If it were diabetes or a heart condition, one could talk openly about it. What is funny is that my best friend Kari and I had been friends since the ninth grade. When I was diagnosed, I didn't tell any of my friends. If they asked, I simply said that I had a digestive disorder. That is why it was so surprising to hear my best friend Kari describe her illness the same way. After one of us finally 'fessed up,' it turned out we both had IBD and she has been my best supporter ever since."

NIKKI, 17

---

inquiries as "gross," not to mention intrusive. While young people are unlikely to totally misrepresent their symptoms, to avoid embarrassing moments, blood tests, or other medical procedures, they may modify their responses. To minimize this sort of evasiveness, parents and physicians should do all they can to persuade children that they are in no way to blame for the illness. Parents and doctors should also ensure that any required tests and procedures are carefully explained and, when administered, accompanied by minimal physical and psychological discomfort. Sedation for unpleasant exams should be adequate.

A physician who enjoys a working dialogue and a rapport with the child can better manage the illness. For this reason, parents should

COLONOSCOPY

"You want me to drink what?" I asked my nurse.

"Don't worry," she said. "It won't hurt you. It just tastes bad."

That was my first encounter with Go-lightly. I took one drink and hoped it would be my last. It seemed like I had to drink what amounted to forty gallons of the stuff to go. In reality, it was only about two more gallons. But still, I couldn't bear drinking it all, so I got the wonderful option of having an NG tube put in. At this point, I was desperate for anything, so I told them sure.

Now remember me saying that the drink's name was Go-lightly? Well, I don't know who came up with this name. I don't think they had an opportunity to sample the product because Go-lightly it is not. It is more like Go-constantly or Go-lots. I'll leave it at that.

Now on to the reason that I had to have the Go-lightly in the first place. It was time for the doctors to get a better look, so they introduced me to the colonoscope. The colonoscope is a device that goes up your bottom to search through your large intestine so the doctors can see where the problem is. After my scope, my doctors said I had what looked like ulcerative colitis."

LIZ, 14

encourage their child to ask questions and to discuss their personal concerns with healthcare providers. You as a parent may be able to help your child be forthright with the doctor by steering the child toward acquiring more information. Most children feel much more in control when they know the facts. One young teenager told her mother that she was able to face her pending surgery without feeling panicky because her mother had always spoken frankly about the illness. On the other hand, it is probably not a good idea to discuss with children the full range of possible complications of IBD, most of which will almost certainly never occur.

Even apparently simple and routine medical procedures such as getting undressed for a physical examination or undergoing a weight check may cause embarrassment or anxiety. Acknowledging these responses, rather than trying to convince children their honest feelings are inappropriate, teaches children that their feelings are respected and deemed worthy of serious consideration by adults. Children, too, have a right to privacy. A child's concerns and choices about who is and who should be in the examining room at any given time should be honored.

Rectal examinations are embarrassing and can be painful if the child has inflammation. Parents or children should feel free to discuss this part of the examination with the doctor if concerns arise. Often, there is little need for the doctor to do a rectal exam on each visit.

Confused by the term "disease," other children, friends, and neighbors may mistakenly believe that IBD is contagious. Parents should explain that, while IBD patients sometimes do contract contagious infections, IBD is not an infection and is not transmissible by personal contact.

Secretly or openly, some adolescents worry about the costs of their medical care and about being a financial burden to the family. They become anxious when a parent is required to miss work to accompany them to a doctor's office or hospital. It is important for parents to be reassuring in this regard by protecting the child from money worries.

Anxieties about slowed growth and sexual development are common. These can be particularly intense for a young woman with low weight. A young woman who does not menstruate when her disease is active should be reassured that her normal menstrual cycle will return as soon as her symptoms are brought into remission and an adequate nutritional regimen reinstated.

Physicians use several approaches to treat impaired growth, weight loss, and delayed sexual maturation. When highly caloric nutritional supplements and protein-enriched drinks do not produce growth, there are other methods of providing nutrition. Nighttime nasogastric tube feedings and intravenous supplementations are sometimes indicated. Face-to-face meetings with other young people who are successfully using

TUBE FEEDINGS

"I first got sick when I was nine years old. I had bad stomachaches and I lost a lot of weight. I was so sick I was sent to a specialist. I had to drink barium for a test and I threw it up. Then I had to have a colonoscopy and all I remember was the nurse saying, 'Rachel, put your head on a pillow.' I still have the pictures from that test. I had to spend five weeks in the hospital with no food. Finally, the doctor let me eat again. Then I had to go back to the hospital for two weeks. No food again. I had to have an NG tube for tube feedings for a long time. I kept the tube in because I didn't like the idea of taking it out and putting it back in every day. Finally, I was able to eat again. But I take lots of medicine all the time."

RACHEL, 11

these techniques often provide a child with the willingness to accept the necessity of these feedings.

Parents can also encourage their children to cope by pointing to examples of people with inflammatory bowel disease who have gone on to live full lives. These might include World War II general and former President, Dwight Eisenhower, Marvin Bush (son of former President George Bush), baseball player Trevor Williams, former place kicker for the San Diego Chargers, Rolph Benirschke, actress Mary Ann Mobley, hockey player Kevin Dineen, and other "ordinary people" from every walk of life. It may also help to introduce your child to members of CCFA who have lived with inflammatory bowel disease since childhood.

Many teenagers are concerned about having inherited IBD. A teenager with a parent who has IBD may harbor a certain amount of anger toward the parent for "passing it on." Obviously, this situation is not helped if anyone else in the household including the other parent seems to share in this resentment. While there does seem to be a genetic predisposition to inherit a susceptibility to IBD, no one has any control over who will actually develop the disease. Similarly, children may worry about "passing the disease on" to their own children. Current information indicates the likelihood of parenting a child with IBD when one parent has IBD is small, about 3% percent (somewhat higher if both parents have IBD). Frank discussions with your gastroenterologist, within the family, and perhaps with a family therapist, can sometimes be helpful in addressing these issues.

Thinking ahead to their lives as more mature adults with a desire to start families of their own, teenagers with inflammatory bowel disease often worry that the disease will interfere with the ability to conceive or enjoy a successful pregnancy. Teens concerned about their eventual childbearing prospects will find it reassuring to know that, with the disease under good control (or even mildly active), most women with IBD will be able to experience a normal pregnancy. Inflammatory bowel disease and its implications for pregnancy are discussed with more detail in chapter 15.

Puffy faces, unwanted fat, acne, and other undesirable side effects can result from corticosteroid medications. While these side effects can sometimes be overwhelming, children taking these medications should be informed that these side effects are temporary and reverse themselves once steroid treatments have been discontinued. Sometimes, corticosteroid-sparing medications such as azathioprine and 6-mercaptopurine may be added to sulfasalazine (5-ASA) or metronidazole in order to reduce the need for heavy steroid doses.

Over and above their physical side effects, medications taken to control inflammatory bowel disease are likely to have some impact on the emotions. Corticosteroids may cause insomnia or produce significant mood swings, particularly in children who were already prone to such emotions prior to diagnosis. Because of this, children should be told in advance that there is some chance that corticosteroids or other medications may make them feel sad or unusually elated. Sulfasalazine, for example, may contribute to depression. The nausea sometimes experienced from metronidazole may diminish a child's sense of well-being. The doctor should be kept advised of any significant mood swings that accompany the use of medications. Tapering or changing the medication, when possible, will resolve many emotional or mental problems. At times, a child who is having trouble in school or in maintaining friendships may be referred to a psychiatrist who may recommend therapy or anti-anxiety medication. A change in physical appearance makes children extremely self-conscious, often arousing feelings of restlessness and moodiness. Unaddressed, such changes may bring on feelings of isolation and the desire to be left alone.

> ## THE VIOLINIST'S SONG
>
> Last year when my strings were
>   broken
> And I was feeling bad,
> Time, patience, and courage
> Were about all I had.
> Made me look like chub,
> "But you have to take it,"
> said Dr. Shub.
> I missed a lot of school,
> And that made me sad;
> At home I was cared for
> By my mom and dad.
> I followed my instructions
> From my nice nurse, Nancy,
> And finally I got better,
> Which suited my fancy.
> And now that my strings
> Are in a state of repair,
> I have a little tune
> That I would like to share.
>
> LISA, 11

Medications can control many symptoms and allow a child to live a more rewarding life. However, it is essential for parents, physicians, teachers, and friends to recognize and share the special concerns of young people with these diseases. The best way to do this, of course, is to talk with them and acknowledge their struggles to improve their lives.

Until about 30 years ago, many physicians believed that emotional factors caused Crohn's disease and ulcerative colitis. Thankfully, as we have learned more about the genetic and immunological processes involved in IBD, there has been a gradual shift from this viewpoint. Today, medical energy is being directed away from seeking information about the supposed psychological makeup of patients and their families and toward treating the diseases, as well as the emotional burdens experienced by young people required to live with them every day.

It is important for children with inflammatory bowel disease and their families to realize that they are not alone in their emotional distress. There are organizations, sources of information, and various support groups created to help children and families diminish the psychological impact of these illnesses. In particular, IBD patients may wish to make contact with the Crohn's & Colitis Foundation of America, Inc. (CCFA) and avail themselves of the many services offered by national and local chapters of this organization (see *About the Crohn's & Colitis Foundation* at the back of the book).

CHAPTER 13

SCHOOL, CAMP, AND PLAY

The intensity of the illness and the personality of the child will understandably factor into family decisions about whether or not to share personal medical information with others. Some families will be forthcoming, while others will feel that almost any personal disclosure outside the family will expose the child to possible embarrassment or discrimination. A child's feelings about sharing and personal privacy should be of paramount importance.

Regardless of your family's policy about sharing information with relatives and friends, clear, regular lines of communication must be observed and maintained with school teachers, nurses, and health personnel. Home and work phone numbers of parents, and the doctor's phone number should be kept up to date and on file in the school health office. This is important because your child is likely to need to

---

THE BOOK SALE

"The way my book sale worked was I had students and staff bring in any used books they had at home. The way I got the word out was by our weekly school news update. The price for each book was fifty cents. Dorey and Daren helped with the sale. It lasted for three days.

"Enclosed you will find a check made out to CCFA for $90.80. This is how much we raised. I would like to put this money toward general research on Crohn's disease.

"The reason why I chose to give you the money is because I have Crohn's disease. My brother and my father and many other people in my family also have it. I think yours is a very worthwhile cause and should have donations made to it."

JEREMY, 12

---

make frequent trips to the bathroom during periods of IBD activity. Ideally, for the sake of privacy and feelings of personal dignity, a child should be given unlimited access to teachers' or nurses' bathrooms.

The fact that your child may require regular medications is another reason for being clear and forthcoming with school authorities. To make matters easier, it may be a good idea to ask your child's doctor to prepare a packet of educational material about IBD for you to provide to nurses and educators. School personnel are usually grateful for the opportunity to become more familiar with sensitive issues confronting children and families with inflammatory bowel disease. Bear in mind that CCFA has developed excellent educational materials for these purposes.

THE SUPPORT OF TEACHERS

Crohn's disease and ulcerative colitis can impair your child's enjoyment of school. Should hospitalization become necessary, your child is likely to miss classes and schoolwork. Tutors can help a child catch up with schoolwork missed due to hospitalization or the need to remain out of school. Under these circumstances, the support and encouragement of teachers and school friends will be indispensable. The support and goodwill of teachers is important for still another reason: teachers and school officials may

> ### THE COMFORT OF CATS
>
> "Daisy, T.K. (Tenacious Kitty), and Binky are my three cats. When I found out that I had ulcerative colitis two years ago my cats were a great comfort to me. I was very sick, stayed in the house most of the time, had no energy, and looked and felt miserable. There were many nights when I would wake up crying because my stomach hurt so much. Now I'm in remission and able to enjoy all the things a kid should. Feeling well makes me very appreciative and thankful. It also makes me very understanding about how people who are always ill must feel."
>
> NATALIE, 12

be the first people to notice that a child is having IBD-related difficulties. Since early intervention is often the key to preventing more extreme or prolonged problems, a regular flow of communication between parents and teachers ought to be encouraged.

A sick child's need for friendship and goodwill cannot be overstated. When hospitalized, many young people appreciate receiving cards, telephone calls, or other forms of communication from classmates.

Teachers and others at school may need to know that Crohn's disease and ulcerative colitis are not caused by emotional stress or diet. As a parent, you may find you have a role in teaching educators, particularly in helping them understand that inflammatory bowel disease symptoms tend to worsen or subside for reasons that are impossible to predict. In addition, the adults with whom your child is in contact at school may need to be told that Crohn's disease and ulcerative colitis are chronic diseases requiring medications which, while they often alleviate the symptoms, do not constitute cures in and of themselves. Adults, teachers, and other children may also need the simple reassurance that Crohn's disease and ulcerative colitis are not contagious.

PHYSICAL EDUCATION

Owing to fluctuations in your child's health, participation in sports and gym may sometimes be undesirable. A note from the doctor to the athletic director of the child's school should make things easier in this regard. Overall, however, it is best that a child with IBD remain active and not become a "couch potato." Children with inactive inflammatory bowel disease have been known to use their illness as an excuse for not participating in sports and other physical activities. This practice should be seriously discouraged. Children should be helped to understand that exercise is a valuable form of rehabilitation and an excellent measure of recovery. For these reasons, young people should be persuaded to participate in sports unless they are experiencing intense symptoms and require high doses of medication. Of course, some strenuous sports may aggravate abdominal pain or joint discomfort and contribute to fatigue in children taking steroids or other medications. In many instances, shorter periods of sports activity may be indicated. Reluctant athletic participants may

---

A DONATION IN FRIENDSHIP

"My name is Scott. It was just my Bar-Mitzvah and I became a man. I received a lot of money and would like to donate to you in honor of my good friend, Aron, who has the illness (IBD). We are very good friends and I sleep over his house a lot and we have loads of fun. We've been friends since we were babies. My friend Aron suffers a lot from his illness. I wanted to do something to help Aron, so I decided to donate some of my money to you so you can try to find a cure."

SCOTT

be inspired to know that more than a few professional athletes have struggled with inflammatory bowel disease. Though the young athlete may need to realize that some strength and endurance skills can be affected by flare-ups of IBD, team sports can be both rewarding and challenging. Even though some children with IBD may need gentle reminders to lower their expectations at times, it is important that they remain as involved as possible in physical activities.

TOILET FACILITIES

Many people with IBD say their most difficult problem in dealing with the disease consists of needing to use the toilet frequently and unpredictably. Attacks of crampy pain and diarrhea often occur without warning. Children with Crohn's disease and ulcerative colitis must have unrestricted freedom to leave the classroom quickly without attracting undue attention. Teachers and school personnel need to understand that questioning the child's need for toilet facilities will cause extreme embarrassment and shame. Any enforced delays may result in a humiliating accident. Unfortunately, in some schools, bathrooms are kept locked for security reasons. Other schools have doorless toilet stalls. Naturally, any accommodation the school can provide to your child which reduces anxiety associated with the need to use the toilet will be of great benefit. Access to a private bathroom in the nurse's office or faculty area is worth working for on behalf of your child.

MEDICATIONS AT SCHOOL

Students with ulcerative colitis and Crohn's disease often need to take medications during the school day in order to help control diarrhea and abdominal cramps. Schools generally require that necessary medications be delivered to the child by the school nurse, and many school districts require written documentation for the medications taken by students. These documents require periodic updating, so parents should stay on top of any such requirements. It is very desirable that arrangements be made for these medicines to be administered unobtrusively. Children should not unnecessarily be made tardy or become the subject of unwanted attention from school friends.

FIELD TRIPS

There is no reason that children with inflammatory bowel disease should be prevented from participating in field trips. Students with IBD and their parents should be informed about these excursions in advance, however, so that medical and toilet facilities can be located and identified before a child goes on the outing. Of course, if the child is experiencing a flare-up of the disease, it may be necessary to travel with the parent in a car or not attend.

AFTER SCHOOL ACTIVITIES

After school activities are valuable to a child or adolescent. Introspective students with inflammatory bowel disease often have to be especially encouraged to stay involved and not use the illness as an excuse for becoming isolated and unhappy. In contrast, many naturally outgoing children with IBD, especially teenagers, seem almost frantic in their efforts to participate in team sports, after school jobs, volunteer work, and the usual socializing activities. Occasionally, as with other children, some limits have to be set.

STANDARDIZED TESTS

Standardized tests such as the SATs can be sources of intense anxiety. Young people with inflammatory bowel disease may postpone or avoid taking these tests because of worries that test performance will be negatively impacted by disease activity. One common source of anxiety to children with inflammatory bowel disease is that they may be required to spend time otherwise allotted for completing a particular school test in the bathroom. By prior arrangement, most tests can be taken "untimed," thereby relieving this particular source of worry.

TRAVEL FROM HOME

In general, a child probably should not travel very far unless the disease is well controlled. Even when symptoms are quiet, travel is a common source of anxiety. The child's anxiety is connected, more often than not, with worries about access to a bathroom. Parents can sometimes be more anxious about this than their children. Children who travel overnight should do so with adult chaperones who have been made fully aware of the child's special needs.

Parents will need to plan carefully when a child is attending summer camp or visiting distant relatives over the summer. When practical, such journeys can provide good training for young people who are likely to be going away to college. For adolescents with IBD, college provides not only the usual academic education, but the opportunity to assume a greater degree of personal responsibility in matters related to health.

DATING AND SOCIALIZATION

When children begin to date, there are issues and adjustments that must be made. However, these illnesses do not necessarily interfere with dating and socialization among adolescents. Although some children will have difficulties, most will adapt themselves to the intense relationships of adolescence. In fact, having struggled long and hard against IBD, many if not most young inflammatory bowel disease patients mature rather quickly and learn to handle social situations extremely well. Children who feel stigmatized by IBD should be recognized early. Counseling and interventions can be very helpful to children facing social difficulties.

CHAPTER 14

FAMILY LIFE

As a parent, you undoubtedly already know a great deal about the difficulty of explaining a serious illness like IBD to your child. At times, you probably feel you could use some help in this important task. A simple rendering of the intestinal tract may do more to help your child understand the illness than a long explanation filled with medical terminology. If your child is young, personal conversations about the illness can be effectively supplemented with pictures, diagrams, and illustrations.

There may be times when your child is intensely curious about the disease and filled with questions. There will almost certainly be times when he or she will not want to talk or think about personal health problems. On still other occasions, a child's curiosity is likely to be both limited and specific. Parents will do well to be aware of the fine line between making themselves available to share, and insisting on long, unwanted discussions. In this respect, a parent can do no better than follow the cues offered by the particular child.

Some children, of course, are older and more detail-minded. Others tend to become anxious, distracted, and forget what they have been told. A child provided with a notebook or journal can be encouraged to write down any questions that arise. Questions that parents find themselves unable to answer can be asked of the doctor at the next scheduled appointment.

Few things are as conducive to anxiety as the unknown. Children with IBD are likely to have to undergo blood tests, as well as a number of other uncomfortable gastrointestinal examinations. Some children will require surgery. By acting as an intermediary and communicating carefully with your child's physician, you can provide information to your child and help the doctor and child communicate effectively. It is important to avoid overwhelming a child with excessive detail. In explaining a procedure, you and the doctor can adjust what is said to a level suited to the child's understanding, personality, and attention span.

A Parent's Concerns

"I love my daughter Julie so much! That thought helps me soothe the hurt and anger I feel knowing there's no cure for IBD. Julie was diagnosed when she was two. Now she is eight. Although she has been stable and off steroids for about a year, continuous flare-ups from a very young age have affected her emotionally and physically. I need to remind myself that the words 'normal child' are a burden for me and a standard set by someone else. Julie deserves to be seen and loved for who she is. There is a place for lectures and explanations about IBD and a child's developmental responses to it, but I also need acknowledgment and support for my powerful desire to help my child and give her what she needs to grow. How much harder that is to do because of her illness!

"For example, tolerating the anxiety over her pain. Tolerating so much 'not knowing.' Is this tantrum a part of a flare-up or is it her age? Tolerating so much helplessness when I can't make things better for her is very difficult. Tolerating patterns of illness, knowing we will have to wait days or weeks until it is appropriate to change dosage or medicine is yet another challenge. Tolerating resistance to taking medication several times a day, every day. Tolerating low eating levels and rising to the challenge of becoming endlessly creative in the administration of food. Tolerating her peers' growth and progress while she will have to wait longer to develop in these ways. Tolerating not knowing when the next flare-up will be.

"Tolerating this disease for the rest of Julie's life. It will take much more than a year of remission for her to catch up with her peers socially and emotionally. Please understand that my heart is still broken and that sometimes it takes many years for a family to heal."

JULIE'S MOTHER

By speaking plainly and being very concrete, you can make the uncertainties of IBD more tolerable for your child.

Families struggling with chronic illness have many common problems. Many share a tendency to become overly involved in the child's illness. Others avoid healthy expressions of anger and other emotions. Parents sometime go too far to protect the child from siblings and peers. While all families are stressed at times, parents with sick children are likely to experience stress levels that fluctuate according to the severity of a child's symptoms. A recent study conducted by CCFA showed that families with Crohn's disease were psychologically less well adjusted than families with ulcerative colitis. Since Crohn's is often more complicated and more seriously debilitating than ulcerative colitis, this finding was, perhaps not all that surprisingly, related to the severity of the child's illness.

ADJUSTING TO LIFE WITH IBD

There are many ways for parents and families to deal with internal pressures in the family. Parents are encouraged to face problems head on by anticipating potential difficulties before they arise. Accept your child's feelings and encourage direct communication about fears and anxieties. Talk matters over with your child's physician. Seek the input of the other parent or, if that's not possible, talk things over with mature adults whose judgment you respect. If it becomes difficult to resolve important issues within the family, don't hesitate to seek professional counseling for yourself, your child, and your family.

Fight feelings of helplessness. Don't force your child into assuming responsibility for the management of the disease, but as signs of

---

SELF-MANAGEMENT

"I am learning that the most important skill we can teach our children with Crohn's disease or ulcerative colitis is self-management. We need to encourage our children to view themselves as people rather than just patients. A comfortable balance in school, leisure, and health activities is essential.

"Stress is 'normal' for teenagers, with or without a chronic disease. At stressful times our parental instincts lead us to 'jump in,' attempt to make things better. Yet if our children are feeling well, we must learn to step back and allow them to have some control over their own lives, as in talking to their doctors and taking their medications. This also helps in developing positive self-esteem and self-sufficiency.

"Over the years, we have taught our children what is important in life. We hope this knowledge will help them consider their own needs and possible limitations. We may make some mistakes, but if our sons and daughters learn self-management skills, they will be allowed to grow and develop into adulthood. This is the greatest gift we can give to our children."

JOYCE, THE MOTHER OF TWO TEENS WITH IBD

maturity develop, do encourage responsible personal decisions about disease care and maintenance. Children encouraged to assume greater control of their own lives gain independence and greater self-confidence. Also, it is important to limit a child's isolation and loneliness. Continued involvement in the daily affairs of the family is important to children with chronic health concerns.

PRESSURE ON SIBLINGS

With varying degrees of justice, sisters and brothers of siblings who are ill often feel that their parents neglect them. Because of this, they sometimes harbor or act out hostile feelings toward the child with IBD. Though you may not be able to avoid such episodes altogether, there are some things that you as a parent can do to minimize family tensions. Require your child with IBD to follow family rules concerning bedtime, chores, allowances, and other matters pertaining to privilege and responsibility within the family. Encourage your sick child to join in family activities and cooperate on an equal footing with brothers and sisters. It is also important to allow *all* your children to express their feelings. Open confrontations and expressions of anger are perfectly normal. Everyone in the family should be encouraged to learn your standards of acceptable and unacceptable behavior and adapt to them. Both adults and children should be allowed to express emotions without undue guilt and shame.

COMMUNICATING WITH FRIENDS AND FAMILY

How much of your child's illness and family stresses you choose to share with less immediate family members or friends is, of course, entirely up to you. While sharing fears and anxieties and experiences can be helpful, it may be well to remember that some people can be pushy or reckless when it comes to offering opinions and unsolicited advice. When those who are ordinarily a little removed from your child's circumstances press their advice, or insist on providing you with disturbing anecdotes and information, remember that no two cases of inflammatory bowel disease are exactly alike. Furthermore, it may be well to remind yourself that there are limits to the value of other people's experience.

DANGER SIGNS

Many children with IBD and their families cope well, while daily life is more of a struggle for others. What is important is understanding that pressures on your child can become very intense.

HE WHO SINGS

"My mom made me get out of bed and take a walk around the hospital floor. I got up, slipped my feet into the disposable slippers the hospital had given me, grabbed my IV Pole, and started out the door. I stepped out into the hallway and then I saw her.

"A little girl with bright red hair and food dribbling down her face was sitting in a high chair, throwing her breakfast everywhere but in her mouth. I started smiling at this little girl who was having so much fun driving the nurses crazy. I turned to the nurse standing next to me and asked why the little girl was in the hospital.

" 'Liver transplant,' she answered curtly.

"Immediately shame overcame me. This little girl having the time of her life was awaiting a liver transplant while I was wallowing in self-pity over having to spend a week of my sophomore year in the hospital.

"As I watched the little girl, I thought of Cervantes' lines. 'He who sings, frightens away his ills.' I realized right then the importance of inner strength. I needed strength to survive my hospital stay and to overcome my illness. I needed to be strong enough to listen to my body when it told me to slow down. I needed to be strong enough not to look at myself as a teenager with a disease but as a teenager who was overcoming an illness. I took one last look at that little girl with red hair and started singing a little song to myself as I turned around and started walking back to my hospital room."

CASSIE, 17

Social isolation and prolonged periods of depression, boredom and listlessness, coupled with a lack of interest in relationships and persistent immature behavior should be regarded as signs that a child is under intense stress and may, in addition to your love and support, need professional counseling. While it is quite natural for children with health problems to pass through difficult periods when they don't feel well, prolonged spells of unhappiness should be addressed by therapeutic professionals outside the family. Often a child's inability to cope with IBD can involve difficult relationships with other family members. For that reason, family counseling can be even more important and productive than individual counseling.

Attention to the needs of patients, parents, siblings, grandparents, relatives and friends is important. Everyone should be allowed to express concerns and anxieties. Open communication is critical for the resolution of conflict. No one is to blame for the illness, but everyone is needed to provide support and nurturing during the years of maturation and physical growth of a child with IBD.

CHAPTER 15

PREGNANCY

Many teenage girls with IBD are concerned about their eventual ability to bear children. It is important to know how pregnancy will affect the course of a patient's disease. In general, women with Crohn's disease or ulcerative colitis seem to conceive as readily as women without IBD. Studies have shown that women with ulcerative colitis have the same rate of fertility as healthy women. Studies of the fertility rates of women with Crohn's disease are conflicting. One large study showed no difference in fertility rates, while older studies and one recent study show a slightly decreased rate of conception in women.

If the male partner is taking sulfasalazine, temporary male infertility may occur. This is because sulfasalazine decreases sperm production, which is a reversible side effect. Before attempting conception, the male partner should stop taking sulfasalazine and/or change to a 5-ASA compound, such as Dipentum®, Asacol®, or Pentasa®, medications which have not been shown to interfere with sperm production.

It is true that any woman contemplating pregnancy should consider the state of her health before conceiving. In fact, it is a good idea for a woman to have her disease in remission before pregnancy. Women with either Crohn's disease or ulcerative colitis should do well during pregnancy if the disease was inactive at the time of conception. If a pregnancy occurs during a period of active disease, however, symptoms of either Crohn's disease or ulcerative colitis are likely to remain active or get worse. This decline in health generally occurs during the first trimester (3 months) in ulcerative colitis, and either during the first trimester or a few months after delivery in Crohn's disease.

If either disease can be brought into remission with drug therapy during the pregnancy, the woman's health should be good for the remainder of the pregnancy.

Pregnant women with IBD have normal deliveries and healthy babies in roughly the same proportions as women in the general population. If there is a problem affecting the pregnancy, it usually occurs in women with active Crohn's disease. These women run a greater risk of premature delivery, stillbirth, or spontaneous abortion. If symptoms become severe enough to require surgery, the risk to the fetus becomes even greater.

There are many reports of ulcerative colitis starting during pregnancy, but recent studies suggest that this time of onset is no more common than any other. Crohn's disease may also begin during pregnancy. Only rarely do these diseases commence during the postpartum period (the weeks immediately following delivery).

In order to avoid any possible harm to the fetus, it is only natural for the pregnant woman and her obstetrician to want to restrict all medications during pregnancy. Sulfasalazine, prednisone, and more recently the 5-ASA compounds (Dipentum®, Asacol®, Pentasa®) are the drugs used most commonly to control the symptoms of Crohn's disease and ulcerative colitis. A recent national study has found no evidence that the fetus is harmed by sulfasalazine or prednisone taken by the mother during pregnancy. And since sulfasalazine is metabolized in the bowel lumen to sulfapyridine and 5-ASA, it is thought that the 5-ASA compounds should be at least as safe as sulfasalazine during pregnancy. Because the major threat to pregnancy appears to come from the active disease itself and not from medications, these drugs should not be discontinued just because a woman becomes pregnant. If either disease worsens severely during the pregnancy, prednisone, sulfasalazine, or a 5-ASA compound may be introduced or increased. Sulfasalazine or a 5-ASA compound may also be used to maintain a remission for the remainder of the pregnancy and after.

SIDE EFFECTS

Sulfasalazine may cause nausea, which adds to the nausea commonly experienced in early pregnancy. The drug may also cause heartburn much like the heartburn sometimes experienced in pregnancies in which there is no IBD.

NURSING

Although some sulfasalazine does pass into the breast milk, its concentration is much reduced and has not been shown to harm the newborn. Five-ASA compounds have not been shown to harm the newborn during nursing. However, there is one report of a nursing baby developing diarrhea following a mother's use of a 5-ASA rectal suppository. The baby's diarrhea stopped when the mother's therapy was discontinued. When clinically feasible, the dosage of prednisone should be reduced and the drug discontinued as quickly as possible in any nursing mother. If a mother wishes to nurse her baby while still taking a moderate or high dose of prednisone, the baby should be monitored carefully by a pediatrician.

IMMUNOSUPPRESSIVES

Studies of animals given immunosuppressive medication while pregnant have found evidence of genetic damage to offspring. Although there are no studies of the genetic effects of these drugs in humans, patients are advised not to become pregnant while taking these medications. A preliminary study from Mt. Sinai suggests that 6-MP may not have serious effects on a fetus. However, additional evaluation is needed to confirm these observations.

DIAGNOSTIC PROCEDURES

Provided they are necessary for diagnosis or management of IBD, examinations such as abdominal ultrasound, sigmoidoscopy, rectal biopsy, upper endoscopy, and colonoscopy are safe in pregnancy. An MRI scan is probably safe, but more information is needed. Diagnostic x-rays should be postponed until after delivery. If a medical emergency necessitates an x-ray, it should be a limited study, and the baby should be shielded.

SURGERY

Whenever possible, surgery should be postponed until after delivery. If the disease is severe and not responding to drug therapy, however, it may be dangerous to the patient not to operate. It is a matter of weighing the risks. Although there are reports of intestinal resections and ileostomies performed successfully in pregnant women, the risk to the fetus is increased when any abdominal surgery is performed.

PREVIOUS SURGERY

In Crohn's disease, previous bowel resection does not appear to affect the pregnancy in any way. In fact, since resection usually results in a remission of symptoms, the patient is likely to do better during the pregnancy than with serious disease symptoms. After ileoanal anastomosis for ulcerative colitis, women have had successful pregnancies. Women with ileostomies for ulcerative colitis or Crohn's disease occasionally suffer prolapse or obstruction of the ileostomy during pregnancy. Because of this, it is best to postpone pregnancy for one year after the ileostomy is constructed (whether conventional or continent ileostomy) to allow the body time to adapt and fully recover from surgery. In Crohn's disease complicated by abscesses or fistulas around the rectum and vagina, episiotomy (standard surgery to widen the birth canal) should be avoided. In these cases, delivery is by Cesarean section.

EARLIER PREGNANCIES

There is no evidence that the course of either disease during any one pregnancy will be the same during any subsequent pregnancies.

INHERITING THE DISEASE

There is a certain risk that a child born to a mother or father with inflammatory bowel disease may develop IBD. However, as has been discussed, IBD is not, strictly speaking, inherited in the same way eye color or some other traits are. Recent studies suggest that the risk to the offspring of developing inflammatory bowel disease if one parent has the disease is about 10%, and if two parents have the disease, as high as 36%. When inflammatory bowel disease clusters in families, there does not seem to be any clear-cut mode of inheritance. Because of this, the diseases are called "familial" and not "genetic." No one can predict whether a child will inherit the disease from his or her parent. It is impossible to predict at what age a child may contract IBD.

DIET

In general, the pregnant woman with Crohn's disease or ulcerative colitis should follow the same well-balanced diet recommended for all pregnant women. The obstetrician and/or gastroenterologist may recommend supplements of specific foods, vitamins, and minerals. If the disease is active, however, it may be necessary to eliminate any foods from the diet that cause discomfort. CCFA's brochure, "Questions and Answers about Diet and Nutrition," contains helpful advice on what foods may cause discomfort.

EMOTIONS AND PREGNANCY

Emotional stress may cause symptoms to worsen during pregnancy, just as stress may do at any other time. This does not mean that stress plays any role in causing the disease, or even that your stress will affect the baby. Similarly, the postpartum period is a time normally characterized by rapid change, both physical and emotional, in the new mother. These changes may also cause a temporary worsening of symptoms.

CHAPTER 16

QUESTIONS AND ANSWERS FOR YOUNG PATIENTS

WHAT ARE CROHN'S DISEASE AND ULCERATIVE COLITIS?

Crohn's disease and ulcerative colitis are diseases of the gastrointestinal (GI) tract. The GI tract works like this: when you eat, food goes down into your stomach. Food leaves the stomach and goes into the small and then the large intestines. In the small intestine, which is a long, winding tube, food is broken down and absorbed by your body. What is left comes out of your bottom as a stool or bowel movement.

Crohn's disease is an illness in which the wall of the intestine becomes sore, inflamed, and swollen. This causes stomachaches, diarrhea (watery stools), fever, weight loss, and blood in your stools. In Crohn's disease, any part of your GI tract, from your mouth to your bottom, may have inflammation. Most commonly, the disease occurs in the last part of the small intestine (called the ileum) or the upper part of the large intestine (called the cecum).

In ulcerative colitis, only the large intestine (colon) is red and swollen. The disease also causes stomach pain and diarrhea, often containing blood. Unlike Crohn's disease, ulcerative colitis does not affect other parts of the GI tract.

Because Crohn's disease and ulcerative colitis inflame the intestines and cause similar symptoms, the two diseases are grouped together under the name inflammatory bowel disease, abbreviated as IBD.

WHAT CAUSES IBD?

We do not know. Most people who study IBD, however, think that your immune system, which normally protects you against disease, may be overworking in the intestine. Instead of protecting your intestine from germs that can make you sick, the immune system may attack your intestine, causing inflammation. We do not know what makes your immune system work too hard and cause IBD, but we do know that IBD is not contagious. No one gave IBD to you, and you cannot give it to anyone else. IBD is not caused by "nerves" or by any kind of food. Nothing that you or your parents ever did caused you to have IBD, so there is absolutely no reason to feel bad or guilty about it.

DOES IBD AFFECT ONLY THE GI TRACT?

Symptoms may also occur outside the gastrointestinal (GI) tract. These include arthritis, mouth ulcers, skin rashes, and eye problems. Arthritis is joint swelling and stiffness. The knees and ankles are most often involved. Swelling usually lasts a few weeks and then disappears with no permanent damage. Controlling the intestinal inflammation will usually fix the joint problems. Small mouth ulcers are like canker sores inside the mouth. They are sometimes present when the bowel is actively inflamed, but they disappear when the inflammation is treated. Sometimes people get skin rashes or painful, reddish bumps on their legs. These get better with treatment of the intestinal inflammation. Eye problems include redness of the eyes, eye pain, or sensitivity to light. These, too, improve with treatment.

CAN IBD EVER BE CURED?

We do not talk about a cure for Crohn's disease or ulcerative colitis, because no one has found one yet. As we have said, we do not even know what causes IBD. You may feel better knowing that many people throughout North America (and the rest of the world) are doing research to find a cure for IBD. Even though we have no cure, there is medicine and there are other things we can do to make you feel better, let you go back to school, and do what you want to do. In some people with severe ulcerative colitis, the disease can be "cured" by removing the colon.

WHAT MEDICINES WILL I HAVE TO TAKE?

Most people take medicine that contains 5-ASA, which is something like aspirin. People may also take prednisone, which is a steroid, or 5-ASA and prednisone at the same time. Some examples of 5-ASA drugs include sulfasalazine (brand name Azulfidine®), Asacol®, Dipentum®, Pentasa®, and Rowasa®. These medicines can be pills, but most of them can be turned into liquids if you do not like to swallow pills.

Sometimes, these medicines can be put into your bottom as solid pellets called suppositories. They can also be mixed in water before going into your bottom; this is called an enema. Sometimes, you have to go into the hospital so that the medicine can be given through a small tube in your vein, called an IV or intravenous tube. You may need IV medicine for IBD if the medicines taken by mouth or in your bottom are not strong enough. Other medicines include antibiotics and immunosuppressives, which are best discussed by your doctor.

WHAT ARE SIDE EFFECTS?

Medicines sometimes do things we do not like; these are called side effects. Medicine for IBD can give you an upset stomach, make your skin break out in rashes, and give you headaches. Prednisone may make you eat more, make your face swollen, slow your growth, and make you feel moody and restless, especially when given in high doses for long periods. You can help control swelling by not adding salt to your foods and by not eating foods high in salt, such as potato chips, pretzels, pizza, and french fries. As the dosage of prednisone is reduced, however, these side effects will go away. You should tell your parents or doctor if you experience side effects. Blood tests will be done to find out if your medicine is working right.

WILL I NEED TO EAT A SPECIAL DIET?

Because it is so important to get enough calories for good growth, your doctor will probably let you eat anything you want to (within reason). But, be smart. Do not eat any food that makes you feel worse. Sometimes raw foods, like salads, or hard foods, like nuts or popcorn, can cause trouble if your intestine happens to be particularly swollen and narrowed, or if your diarrhea has been worse recently.

WHAT IF I FEEL TOO SICK TO EAT?

If you are having a lot of stomach pain, diarrhea, or bleeding, and medicine is not helping enough, you may not feel like eating. If you do not want regular foods, there are special liquids that you can drink. These often contain everything your body needs and come in many flavors, like vanilla and chocolate. If you cannot drink the special formulas, sometimes it is necessary to put the liquid through a thin soft tube that can be passed through your nose into your stomach. Such a tube is called a nasogastric or an NG tube. This can be done while you are asleep at night. Other times, you may be sick enough to be in the hospital. There, nutrition may be given to you in a liquid going through an IV. Giving nutrition this way is called total parenteral nutrition or TPN. Not everyone needs these special kinds of liquid diets. Your doctor knows that eating more food will help your body fight the disease better.

PLAYING SOFTBALL

"Since I've had Crohn's disease, I've learned to take medicine and nutritional supplements and to watch my diet. I'm having a great year and plan to play softball in the spring."

AMELIA, 9

WILL IBD MAKE ME GROW MORE SLOWLY?

It might, for a while. If you became sick as a young child, you may now be shorter than others in your class. This may be because the IBD slows down your growth or makes you less hungry. If you do not eat enough, you will not grow as fast as you could.

WILL I HAVE TO TAKE MORE TESTS?

If you become sick and your doctor needs to find out what is wrong, you may have to take more tests. You may already know what a barium x-ray is. Barium is a chalky liquid, which you drink, and makes your intestines show up on an x-ray known as an upper GI. A barium enema means that the barium is put in your bottom through a tube. Barium x-rays let your doctor see how sore your intestine is and whether it is getting better with medicine. The other way to see the intestine is by doing an endoscopy. An endoscope is a bendable tube with a bright light and a tiny TV camera at its tip that allows the doctor to see the inside lining of your intestine. The endoscope may go down your throat or into your bottom. Usually, the endoscopy is not done while you are awake. Instead, you get medicine through an IV or a gas mask on your face to make you sleepy. That way, you will not be scared or worried during the test. Later, you may have a hard time even remembering the test. For the endoscopy through your mouth, you must have an empty stomach, which means skipping a meal. For the barium enema or the endoscope through your bottom, stools in your colon need to be cleaned out. This means drinking a lot of clear liquids, eating jello and popsicles for a day or two before the test, and taking laxatives for a few days or drinking a special solution to "flush out" your intestines the night before the test. These tests are not fun. But they may be the only way your doctor can tell which part of your intestine is sore and what the best medicine is to make it better.

WILL I HAVE TO HAVE AN OPERATION?

Surgery is not usually the first way to make you get better. Your doctor may decide you need surgery if the medicines prescribed for you do not work. That is why it is so important for you to take all your medicine.

In Crohn's disease, the surgeon usually removes the inflamed part of the intestine and sews the healthy parts together. This is not a cure for Crohn's disease because the disease often comes back in a different part of the intestine after the operation.

If surgery becomes necessary for ulcerative colitis, all or most of the large intestine is removed. While healing is going on inside, your intestine may temporarily drain the stool through an opening in the front next to your belly button. This is called a stoma or ostomy. The liquid stool is caught in a disposable bag or pouch that sticks to your body with a special glue. Having a stoma sounds bad, but people do get used to it. Usually, stomas are for a short time. After you have healed, you may be reconnected on the inside with more surgery, so you can start to have bowel movements out of your bottom again. When you are reconnected, the stoma is not needed, so it is closed.

WHAT CAN I DO TO MAKE MYSELF FEEL BETTER?

Some people who get sick think the doctors and nurses will make them well. IBD is different. If you have IBD, you will get well only if you work with your doctors and nurses. These are the things you will need to do. Take all your medicine and tell your mom or dad if you think the medicine is making you worse, not better. Pay attention to how much pain you're having and what your bowel movements look like, how watery they are, and how much blood they have. Remember, if you take your medicine, you will feel better.

IS THERE ANY WAY I CAN GET USED TO HAVING IBD?

IBD will be with you off and on for many years. You might feel that you spend too much time thinking about taking your medicine and about bowel movements. The medicine may make you feel and look different. There are times when you may be having more pain and stools and you want your mom and dad to take care of you. But, once you start feeling better, you will want to take care of yourself again.

Sometimes, it helps to tell a friend about your feelings. That way, someone you like understands what you are going through. Your doctor, or nurse, or a specialist called a psychologist, or a counselor may be able to help. Your school nurse and teachers may also be able to understand if they know more about IBD. You, as well as your parents, can tell them how you feel. You may be able to get permission to leave the classroom to use the bathroom without asking every time. People with IBD often keep personal calendars to help them remember their medicine. If you do things like that, you are taking control over the IBD and assuming responsibility for your own body.

CAN I GO TO SCHOOL AND TAKE PART IN SPORTS?

You should do anything you feel like doing. You can play in sports if you feel well enough and if your doctor permits it. On days when you do not feel well, you should not feel guilty about staying home until you feel better. Maybe your teachers and doctor can work out something special just for you.

REMISSION

"I was seven years old when it happened. I would get terrible stomach cramps. I would double over and didn't care where I was. My parents rushed me to the doctor and he said it was all in my mind. My mom took me for a second opinion. They ran all sorts of tests on me and diagnosed me with Crohn's. I was put on all different types of medications. Some made me look fat. Others stunted my growth. I had tube feedings for a couple of months. My mom decided to change doctors. My new doctor took me off the other medication and put me on new ones. These new medicines seem to be working much better. I've been in remission for a while. I'm thirteen and I was just taught how to put my own NG tube in and to do my own tube feedings at night for ten hours. Sometimes I don't feel like I have my illness. I learned to live with my illness. I can drink and eat anything I want. No one suspects me of having my illness. I look like a normal teenager. Hopefully one day they will find a cure."

A YOUNG PATIENT

RESOURCES

ABOUT THE CROHN'S & COLITIS FOUNDATION OF AMERICA

The Crohn's & Colitis Foundation of America (CCFA) is the only national nonprofit organization in America devoted exclusively to inflammatory bowel disease and those who struggle with it. CCFA was established in 1967 and has become a major force among American voluntary health agencies, with 70 nationwide affiliates and more than 130,000 members, donors, and friends. Supported solely through individual, foundation, and corporate contributions, CCFA proudly spends nearly 80 cents of every dollar received on its threefold mission:

1. To support basic and clinical scientific research to find the cause of, and cure for, Crohn's disease and ulcerative colitis.

   CCFA has awarded grants to the foremost IBD researchers in the United States and abroad, and has nurtured the careers of many gifted young researchers. Over the years research has led to many improvements in the diagnosis and treatment of these diseases. Eventually the efforts of researchers may provide us with knowledge of what causes these diseases.

2. To provide educational programs for patients and their families, as well as for medical professionals and the general public.

   In financial reports submitted by voluntary health agencies in the United States, CCFA has consistently ranked higher than most other national health organizations in its percentage allocation of program dollars to public and professional education. CCFA's seminars, books, brochures, and newsletters provide vital information to the public.

3. To offer supportive services for patients, their families, and friends.

   CCFA chapters throughout the country provide support groups and hospital visitation programs designed to help patients cope with ulcerative colitis and Crohn's disease. These programs do a great deal to improve the quality of life of patients and their families.

MEMBERSHIP PROGRAM

CCFA offers memberships to patients and laypersons, physicians, nurses, dietitians, and other medical professionals. Members enjoy the satisfaction and knowledge that they are supporting the foundation's research mission. Additionally, they are able to take advantage of special offers, various educational opportunities, and supportive services. Patient members receive CCFA's national magazine, *Foundation Focus,* along with chapter newsletters, book discounts, and invitations to area events and support programs. Medical professional members receive book discounts, *Foundation Focus*, patient educational packages for distribution, and an annual listing in the *CCFA Healthcare Professionals Roster*. Physician members receive *Foundation Focus*, a discount on CCFA's Medical Journal *Inflammatory Bowel Diseases*, free supplies of CCFA's educational brochures for their patients, and an annual listing in the *CCFA Physicians Roster*. This roster is a valuable referral source for national and chapter offices. Physicians also receive discounts on books and registration fees for CCFA-sponsored professional education workshops. CCFA has created a powerful partnership of laypersons, physicians, and medical professionals who are resolved to conquer Crohn's disease and ulcerative colitis, and we urge you to become part of the solution by joining us.

EDUCATIONAL RESOURCES

Each year, CCFA distributes thousands of educational brochures to patients, hospitals, physicians, medical professionals, and the general public. Each brochure covers a specific topic related to IBD. Diet and nutrition, complications, emotional factors, pregnancy, surgery, children and teenagers, and the school teacher's role, are but a few of the topics that have been treated to date. A general brochure about IBD is also published in Spanish. All brochures are free upon request.

The foundation also offers books about IBD. CCFA members may purchase the following books at a discount:

Treating IBD: A Patient's Guide to the Medical and Surgical Management of Inflammatory Bowel Disease provides the latest information on the medical and surgical treatment of IBD, including the new drug therapies, advances in nutritional care, and recently developed alternatives in surgery.

The New *People...Not Patients: A Source Book for Living with IBD* is the second edition of CCFA's best-selling reference guide. Completely revised with new charts and diagrams, it provides essential information patients need to cope with Crohn's disease or ulcerative colitis. Included is up-to-date information on diagnostic tests, dosages and side effects of IBD medications, together with strategies for coping with ostomies and the new pull-through operations for ulcerative colitis. Employment and insurance problems are among the many subjects covered in the book's 22 chapters.

Foundation Focus, CCFA's national magazine published three times a year offers important news on health and medicine, special feature stories on coping with Crohn's disease and ulcerative colitis, and in-depth information on the research and treatment of these diseases. All CCFA members receive this magazine.

SUPPORTIVE SERVICES

CCFA chapters afford members the opportunity to benefit from several types of educational and supportive services. Educational programs led by prominent physicians and medical professionals are routinely scheduled by local chapters in order to bring audiences the latest information on treatment and research.

Self-help or mutual support groups formed by many CCFA chapters provide patients, parents, families, and spouses, with ideas, friendship, open communication, understanding and trust. In these groups, members are encouraged to discuss their physical problems as well as their fears, anxieties, and the emotional difficulties associated with living with IBD.

Trained volunteers offer emotional support and information about IBD to patients and families through a variety of visitation programs. These services are available through CCFA chapters to people at home or in the hospital.

CCFA is committed to educating the public about IBD and the services which the foundation offers. Chapter staff and volunteers take every opportunity to address local groups, schools, and community functions. The national office administers a speakers bureau featuring well-known athletes and celebrities. Television and radio public service announcements are produced for local and national use. These ongoing efforts in communication have helped CCFA reach out to countless persons affected by IBD and raise thousands of dollars for medical research.

CCFA CAN HELP

Crohn's disease and ulcerative colitis are painful and difficult diseases to live with. Not long ago, people with IBD were fearful of asking questions and were expected to be satisfied with the minimal information they were given. Today, patient education is a priority among physicians and patients alike. While pursuing its ultimate goal of solving the riddles of IBD, the foundation encourages patients and their families to look to CCFA for information and support.

Patients can help themselves by sharing insights and experiences with others. Getting involved as a volunteer promotes well-being. Happily, CCFA is rich in volunteer opportunities for patients and families.

The foundation views its active partnership of laypersons, physicians, and professional staff as the force that will finally conquer IBD. CCFA's goal is nothing less than reaching out to every man, woman, and child in America who suffers from IBD — and to every medical professional responsible for caring for IBD patients. To find out how CCFA can help you, or how you can help yourself while helping CCFA, please call (800) 932-2423 or (212) 685-3440. You can fax us at (212) 779-4098, or write to *Crohn's & Colitis Foundation of America, Inc., National Headquarters, 386 Park Avenue South, 17th Floor, New York, NY 10016-8804.*

BARBARA T. BOYLE
NATIONAL EXECUTIVE DIRECTOR, CCFA

THE NATIONAL DIGESTIVE DISEASES INFORMATION CLEARINGHOUSE

The National Digestive Diseases Information Clearinghouse (NDDIC) is a service of the National Institute of Diabetes and Digestive and Kidney Diseases, part of the National Institutes of Health, under the U.S. Public Health Service. The clearinghouse, authorized by Congress in 1980, provides information about digestive diseases and health to people with these disorders and their families, to medical professionals, and to the public. The NDDIC answers inquiries, develops, reviews and distributes publications, works closely with professional and patient organizations and government agencies, and disseminates accurate, up-to-date information about digestive diseases. For additional information, contact the *NDDIC, 2 Information Way, Bethesda, MD 20892-3570,* or phone (310) 654-3810.

A GUIDE TO IBD MEDICATIONS

This guide is intended to provide readers with some very basic information about medications commonly used in the treatment of inflammatory bowel disease (IBD). Specific questions about any of the medications described in this guide should be referred to a qualified medical doctor experienced in administering and monitoring these medications.

For the sake of brevity, the medicines described in this guide are considered individually. However, any patient being treated for IBD might well take more than one of these medications, and any medication taken in combination with another might produce results or effects which differ significantly from those described in this guide. It is important to understand that the effectiveness of any medication, as well as its potential side effects, may be altered when it is taken in combination with other medicines. For that reason, the patient's physician should be made aware of all medicines being taken; this applies to prescription and nonprescription drugs alike.

Possible side effects associated with individual medications are described below. Many milder side effects subside after a few days or after a medication is discontinued. In fact, most side effects are rare and occur in only a small percentage of patients taking a particular medication. Because of their more potentially serious character, mention is also made of side effects which are rarer still. *That said, we add that if you or your child seems to be experiencing a side effect from a medication, consult the physician who prescribed the medicine immediately.*

Some medications detailed below should not be taken when a patient is pregnant or breastfeeding. Pregnant patients or those contemplating pregnancy will want to communicate closely with doctors about any and all medicines being taken to control IBD.

It is essential to keep all medications stored and labeled in containers provided by the pharmacy, and well out of the reach of children. Do not store medications in the bathroom medicine cabinet where natural heat or moisture might reduce their effectiveness. Dispose of medicines no longer being taken and medicines bearing expired dates. Consult your physician about the proper disposal of unused medications.

Medicines come in different dosages. Before beginning any new medication, patients should consult their doctors about what they should do if a prescribed medicine comes in dosages larger or smaller than those originally called for. Doctors should also be asked about tardiness: some "missed" medicines require the patient to take an extra dose; others do not.

Any medication can trigger an allergic reaction. Symptoms include rashes, hives, wheezing, and shortness of breath. Notify the doctor promptly should any of these reactions begin to occur. Shortness of breath is particularly serious. If a patient is having difficulty breathing, call 911 or activate the emergency medical system in your area.

AZATHIOPRINE (Imuran®)

Reasons for recommending this medication: Azathioprine controls disease activity by suppressing the body's immune response. This medication is sometimes used to help keep IBD in remission while steroids are decreased or discontinued. It is sometimes used as a substitute for steroids and is almost identical to 6-mercaptopurine.

Possible side effects: Hair loss, joint pain, skin rash, loss of appetite, blood disorders, dry mouth, rapid heartbeat, changes in vision, fatigue, pancreatitis, nausea and vomiting, cough, dizziness, sore throat, fever, unusual bleeding or bruising, and yellowing of the skin or whites of the eyes.

Special considerations: This medication should be taken with food to decrease the possibility of developing an upset stomach. Vaccinations, other immunizations, or skin tests should not be taken while a patient is being treated with azathioprine unless specifically authorized by the attending physician. Notify the physician if, while taking this medication, a patient is exposed to the chicken pox or other contagious diseases. Chewing gum or sucking on candy may be helpful to eliminate a dry mouth. It is important to keep all doctors' appointments and laboratory tests while taking this medication. The use of azathioprine during pregnancy may result in harm to an unborn child. Doctors should be consulted by any patient taking this medication contemplating pregnancy. This medication may not become fully effective until after it has been taken for several months.

FERROUS SULFATE (Iron) (Feosol®)

Reasons for recommending this medication: Ferrous sulfate is used to correct or prevent iron deficiency. Iron deficiency in IBD can occur because of blood losses or because the diseased intestine cannot properly absorb the iron naturally present in foods.

Possible side effects: Constipation, diarrhea, nausea, abdominal pain, dark stools, chest or throat pain when swallowing tablets, staining of teeth (when taken in liquid form only).

Special considerations: Keep this medication out of reach of children. *Overdoses can be fatal.* Patients should not take more of this medication than prescribed by doctors. *Immediate medical attention is critically important to a patient who has taken an overdose of this medication. Call your poison control center or nearest emergency room at once.* Store this medication in a cool, dark place. Discoloration of stool is harmless and normal for those taking iron supplements. Notify doctors if this symptom is accompanied by abdominal pain or red streaks in the stool. Take on an empty stomach or with water or juice. Take after meals if stomach upset occurs. Avoid taking antacids or tetracycline in conjunction with iron. Allow 1-2 hours between taking iron and antacid or tetracycline. Mix liquid iron preparations with water or juice to prevent staining of teeth. Brush teeth immediately after taking liquid iron preparations. Iron supplements can lead to the appearance of blood in the stools where none has appeared before.

FOLIC ACID (Folvite®)

Reasons for recommending this medication: Folic acid is used to correct or prevent folic acid deficiency. This deficiency in IBD can occur because the diseased intestine cannot properly absorb folic acid normally found in some foods. It can also occur when sulfasalazine is being taken.

Possible side effects: Skin rash, itching, dark yellow discoloration of urine, difficulty in breathing.

Special considerations: Store in a cool, dark place. Keep all appointments with doctors and laboratories so that patient responses to this medication may be carefully monitored. Discoloration of urine is harmless.

HYDROCORTISONE ENEMAS (Cortenema®)

Reasons for recommending this medication: Hydrocortisone enemas can reduce inflammation in the rectum, sigmoid colon, and descending colon (distal disease). They tend to work quickly and effectively without the risks of side effects associated with oral prednisone.

Possible side effects: (only in cases involving significant systemic absorption) Decreased appetite, increased appetite, stomach irritations, nausea and vomiting, insomnia, vision problems, headaches, dizziness, high blood pressure, night sweats, mood swings, increased sweating, skin irritations, easy bruising, weight gain, fluid retention, increased tendency to develop infections, acne.

Possible long-term side effects: (only in cases of significant systemic absorption) Impaired healing of wounds, muscle weakness, striae ("stretch marks"), elevated blood sugar levels, slowed growth in children, bone fractures, osteoporosis, increased hair growth, irregular menstrual periods, cataracts.

Special considerations: The side effects listed are the same as those listed for oral prednisone. This form of the medication is not absorbed by the body as completely as the oral form. However, side effects are less common with the use of hydrocortisone enemas than with oral prednisone. Carefully read and follow directions. Be sure the doctors know the names of all medications being taken by the patient prior to starting these enemas. Each bottle contains one dose. Use it all unless the doctor indicates otherwise. *Do not discontinue the use of this medication without consulting your doctor. Abrupt withdrawal of this medication can result in serious illness, life-threatening problems, or death.* Notify doctors if there is rectal bleeding, pain, burning, itching, blistering, or if irritations develop which were not present before beginning this medication. *Tell every doctor, dentist, or surgeon responsible for patient treatment about these enemas if they have been taken within a year's time.* Patients using hydrocortisone enemas may require special care in emergency situations. For this reason, it is strongly recommended that patients using this medication carry a medical identification card or wear ID jewelry stating that they are taking this medication or have taken this medication at some point during the past year. Best results are obtained when this medication is used immediately after bowel movements. To best enable the medicine to do its work, patients should lie on the left side for 30 minutes after the enema is given. If possible, the enema solution should be kept in all night.

Possible medication interactions: Few children will be taking these medications. Chlorpropamide, tolbutamide (Diabinese® or Orinase®) or other oral medications used to lower the blood sugar may not be as effective in lowering blood sugar when these enemas are being taken. Warfarin (Coumadin®) is a blood-thinning medication. Its blood-thinning effects can be intensified, meaning the patient runs an increased risk of excessive bleeding when these enemas are being taken.

LOPERAMIDE (Imodium®, Imodium AD®)

Reasons for recommending this medication: Loperamide decreases the number of stools.

Possible side effects: Constipation, nausea, abdominal pain, bloating, dry mouth, fever, rashes, drowsiness, dizziness.

Special considerations: Although this medication is available without a prescription, IBD patients should take it only when recommended by doctors. Do not allow this medication to become frozen. Children taking this medication regularly for a long period of time should be evaluated by doctors for progress at regular intervals. Chewing gum or sucking on hard candy may alleviate a dry mouth. Patients who become drowsy on this medication should not operate a motor vehicle or dangerous machinery. Children taking this medication should be prevented from engaging in bicycle riding or performing other activities requiring good physical coordination.

MERCAPTOPURINE (6-MP, Purinethol®)

Reasons for recommending this medication: Mercaptopurine controls disease activity by suppressing the body's immune response. This medication is sometimes used to keep the disease in remission while steroids are decreased or discontinued. This medication is sometimes used instead of steroids.

Possible side effects: Weakness, chills, headache, sore throat, mouth pain, loss of appetite, blood disorders, dry mouth, pancreatitis, rashes, unusual bleeding, yellowing of the skin or whites of eyes, shortness of breath, nausea and vomiting, cough, dizziness.

Special considerations: To reduce the risk of nausea, patients should take this medication with food. Patients taking this medication should avoid having vaccinations, other immunizations, or skin tests unless the attending physician specifically authorizes them. Notify the physician if the patient has been exposed to chicken pox or any other contagious diseases while being treated with this medicine. Chewing gum or sucking on candy may be helpful in alleviating a dry mouth. It is important to keep doctors' appointments and undergo all scheduled laboratory tests while taking this medication. This medication during pregnancy may result in harm to the unborn child. Consult with doctors about the advisability of pregnancy when taking this medication. Several months usage may be necessary for this medication to become fully effective.

MESALAMINE (oral) (Asacol®, Pentasa®)

Reasons for recommending this medication: Mesalamine helps to reduce inflammation in the intestine. Doctors may choose a form of mesalamine because of the location of a patient's disease. Mesalamine may be used by patients who have experienced allergic reactions to sulfasalazine.

Possible side effects: Abdominal pain, bloating, increased symptoms of colitis, diarrhea, constipation, nausea, gas, weakness, dizziness, fever, headache, sore throat, rashes, itching, back pain, renal (kidney) impairment, pancreatitis, blood disorders.

Special considerations: Swallow tablets or capsules whole, taking care not to break the outer coating. Some patients taking Asacol® report passing the entire tablet in stools. However, it sometimes happens that only the shell is present. If the medication and the shell are passed, it should be reported to the doctor. It is important to keep all doctors' appointments and undergo all scheduled laboratory tests while taking this medication.

MESALAMINE (suppositories or enemas) (Rowasa®)

Reasons for recommending this medication: This medication helps reduce inflammation in the rectum, sigmoid colon and descending colon ("distal disease"). These medications can be used as an alternative or in addition to oral medications.

Possible side effects: Abdominal pain, bloating, increased symptoms of colitis, diarrhea, gas, nausea, dizziness, headache.

Special considerations: (*Suppositories)* Be sure to remove the foil wrapper before using the suppository. Avoid excessive handling of the suppository, which is designed to melt at body temperature. To achieve the best possible results from the suppository, it should be kept in the rectum for 1- 3 hours after insertion. *(Enemas)* Shake the bottle well to make sure the ingredients are thoroughly mixed. Use the enema right before bedtime. To achieve the best possible results from the enema, it should be kept in the rectum for about 8 hours. Each bottle contains a single dose. Use all the medication in the container unless the doctor instructs otherwise.

METRONIDAZOLE (Flagyl®)

Reasons for recommending this medication: Metronidazole is an antibiotic which may be helpful in treating complications of Crohn's disease.

Possible side effects: Nausea, decreased appetite, dry mouth, metallic taste, dark or reddish brown urine, furry tongue, numbness or tingling of the hands and feet, rashes, itching, fever, joint pain, painful urination, weakness, insomnia, headache, dizziness, seizures (with high dosage).

Special considerations: To reduce the risk of an upset stomach take this medication with food. Reddish brown coloration of the urine is not harmful. *Avoid alcoholic beverages and medications containing alcohol.* Use of alcoholic beverages while taking this medication can cause nausea, vomiting, sweating, headache, and flushing. Chewing gum or sucking on hard candy may alleviate dry mouth or unpleasant metallic taste.

Possible medication interactions: Warfarin (Coumadin®) is a blood-thinning medication. Its blood-thinning effect can be increased by metronidazole, resulting in an increased risk of bleeding. The doctor should be told about all other medications being taken.

OLSALAZINE SODIUM (Dipentum®)

Reasons for recommending this medication: Olsalazine helps to reduce inflammation in the colon. This medication may be used in most patients who are allergic to sulfasalazine.

Possible side effects: Diarrhea, worsening of symptoms of colitis, abdominal pain, nausea, decreased appetite, headache, dizziness, fatigue, rash, itching.

Special considerations: To reduce the risk of nausea take this medication with food. Doses of this medication should be evenly spaced throughout the day. Tell your doctor if diarrhea occurs.

PREDNISONE (Deltasone®, Liqui Pred®, Orasone®, Sterapred®, Panasol®)

Reasons for recommending this medication: Prednisone reduces the body's inflammatory response. It is usually very effective and works quickly. Prednisone is generally recommended when IBD symptoms flare up, as well as when the disease is first diagnosed. The goal of prednisone therapy is to put the disease into remission as quickly as possible. The dosage is then lowered and the medication eventually discontinued.

Possible side effects: Increased appetite, stomach irritation, nausea, vomiting, insomnia, vision problems, headache, dizziness, high blood pressure, night sweats, mood swings, increased sweating, skin irritation, easy bruising, weight gain, fluid retention, increased tendency toward infections, acne.

Possible long-term side effects: Impaired wound healing, muscle weakness, striae ("stretch marks"), elevated blood sugar levels, slowed growth in children, bone fracture susceptibility, osteoporosis, increased hair growth, irregular menstrual periods, cataracts.

Special considerations: Do not discontinue this medication without consulting your doctor. Sudden discontinuation of this medicine can result in sickness, life-threatening problems, or death. This medication should be taken with meals or snacks to prevent upset stomachs. This medication should not be taken with other medicines containing alcohol. People taking prednisone require special care in emergency situations. Patients should carry medical identification cards or wear ID jewelry stating that the patient is taking this medication or has taken it in the past year. *Doctors, dentists, surgeons should be aware that the patient is taking prednisone or has taken it within the last year.* Single, daily, or alternate-day doses should be taken in the morning prior to 9:00 am, unless the doctor advises otherwise. Other doses should be spaced evenly throughout the day. Patients should avoid vaccinations, other immunizations, or skin tests unless specifically instructed to the contrary by doctors. Patients exposed to chicken pox or other contagious diseases while taking prednisone should notify their doctor. Store this medication away from heat and light. A low-sodium diet while taking this medication may reduce weight gain associated with water retention. Patients should keep all appointments with doctors and undergo all scheduled laboratory tests so the effects of this medication can be carefully monitored. Growing children taking prednisone should be carefully monitored.

Possible medication interactions: Although rarely taken by IBD patients, chlorpropamide, tolbutamide (Diabinese® or Orinase®) or other oral medications used to lower blood sugar levels may not be as effective in patients taking prednisone and can result in blood sugar elevations. Warfarin (Coumadin®) is a blood-thinning medication. Its blood-thinning effect can be increased by prednisone, resulting in an increased risk of bleeding. Be sure doctors are aware of all other medications being taken.

SULFASALAZINE (Azulfidine®, Azulfidine EN-tabs®)

Reasons for recommending this medication: Sulfasalazine helps reduce inflammation in the colon.

Possible side effects: Diarrhea, headache, loss of appetite, skin rashes, hives, itching, male infertility, yellowish-orange discoloration of urine, blood disorders, sensitivity to light, unusual bleeding or bruising, blood in the urine.

Special considerations: Medication should be taken after meals or with food to reduce risks of nausea. Tablets should be swallowed whole and should not be broken or crushed unless otherwise directed by doctors. Parents of small children are often directed to crush the pill into food or drinks provided to the child. Each dose of sulfasalazine should be accompanied by a full glass of water. Several additional glasses of water should be consumed throughout the day. Yellowish orange discoloration of the urine is harmless. Sulfasalazine increases sensitivity to light. Prolonged exposure to sunlight should be avoided. Protective clothing and sunscreens should be used. Sunlamps should not be used. Because heat and moisture may reduce the effectiveness of this medicine, do not store in the bathroom medicine cabinet. Patients taking this medication should keep all appointments with doctors and undergo all scheduled laboratory tests, so the progress of a patient can be carefully monitored.

Possible medication interactions: The following medications are rarely used in treating IBD, though it is possible they may be taken by patients being treated for other conditions. Chlorpropamide, tolbutamide (Diabinese®, or Orinase®) or other oral medications used to lower blood sugar may be less effective when taking sulfasalazine, resulting in lowered blood sugar levels. Warfarin (Coumadin®) is a blood-thinning medication. Its thinning properties may be increased by sulfasalazine, resulting in an increased risk of excessive bleeding. Digoxin (Lanoxin®), a heart medication, may not be absorbed properly with sulfasalazine, resulting in blood levels that are too low. Phenytoin (Dilantin®), used to control seizures, can work differently when a patient is taking sulfasalazine. Levels of dilantin in the blood can become dangerously high. Doctors should be informed about all medications being taken by a patient who is beginning sulfasalazine.

GLOSSARY OF IBD TERMS

Abscess

A localized collection of pus. Abcesses may form in the abdominal cavity or in the rectal areas of Crohn's disease patients.

Anastomosis

A surgical connection.

Anemia

A blood-related condition characterized by abnormally low amounts of hemoglobin and red blood cells.

Ankylosing spondylitis

A chronic inflammatory disease of the spine and adjacent joints found in some persons with Crohn's disease or ulcerative colitis. The disease affects more males than females, usually occurs in patients under 30, and causes pain and stiffness in the joints of the spine, hips, neck, jaw, and ribcage. Anti-inflammatory drugs, physical therapy, and occasionally surgery are used in treatment.

Aphthous ulcers

Small whitish, painful ulcers, commonly known as cankers, which may occur in the mouth with the onset of IBD symptoms. They appear similar to the early lesions of Crohn's disease sometimes found in the colon.

Arthralgia

Pains in the joints frequently experienced by people with IBD.

Arthritis

Swelling and pain involving one or more joints that may be experienced by persons with IBD, especially those with colon involvement.

Barium enema

An X-ray examination of the colon performed after liquid barium has been used to coat the lining of the rectum. The purpose of the barium is to coat the colon, making it visible to X-rays.

Biopsy

A small piece of tissue taken from the body for purposes of examinination under a microscope. Biopsies are routinely obtained from the inner lining of the GI tract and may be useful in diagnosing IBD. Biopsies are also employed to monitor the progress of medications being taken to alleviate the symptoms of these diseases. Biopsies may also be employed to look for the development of cancer cells, particularly in persons who have had ulcerative colitis more than 10 years.

Breath test
Tests in which air from the breath is analyzed. Breath tests are often done to look for evidence of lactose intolerance, an absence of the enzyme required to digest milk sugar.

Colectomy
Surgical removal of the colon. See proctocolectomy.

Colonoscopy
A test in which a flexible, lighted tube is inserted through the rectum to examine the colon. Biopsies may be taken as a part of this test. Sedatives are usually given to make this procedure more tolerable.

Colostomy
A surgical opening of the colon on the abdominal wall enabling liquid fecal waste to collect in a bag or pouch. A colostomy is done to bypass diseased or surgically removed colon.

Computerized tomography
Also known as a CT scan. A test in which an X-ray machine takes many images of a region of the body from different angles. A computer is used to assemble all the pictures into complete images of internal organs.

Contagious
Communicable; transmissible by contact with the sick or exposure to their fresh secretions or excretions.

Continent ileostomy
The surgical creation of an ileal pouch inside the lower abdomen to collect fecal waste after colectomy for ulcerative colitis. No appliance is required. The pouch is emptied regularly with a small tube inserted through a nipple opening in the lower front part of the abdomen.

Distention
An uncomfortable feeling of swelling in the abdomen often caused by excessive amounts of gas and fluid in the intestine. Severe distention may be a sign of intestinal obstruction or blockage.

Edema
Accumulation of excessive amounts of fluid in the tissues, resulting in swelling.

Elemental diet
Medically prescribed nutrition provided to IBD patients in the form of pre-digested liquids containing all necessary nutrients. These preparations are used to help IBD patients gain weight and sometimes to assist in the healing of intestinal inflammation during disease flare-ups.

Endoscopy
A general term referring to the examination of digestive organs with the help of a lighted tube inserted into the body. The types of endoscopy most often associated with IBD are esophagogastroduodenoscopy (upper endoscopy), colonoscopy, and sigmoidoscopy (lower endoscopy).

Enema
The injection of a liquid into the rectum for cleansing or therapeutic purposes.

Episcleritis
The inflammation of the episclera or "white" of the eye.

Erythema nodosum
Red tender swellings on the lower legs occasionally seen during flare-ups of IBD. Although these lesions are indications of disease activity, they usually subside without a trace when the disease is treated.

Exacerbation
A worsening of symptoms or an increase in disease activity, also known as a relapse or flare-up.

Fissure
A crack in the skin, usually in the area of the anus in Crohn's disease.

Fistula
An abnormal inflamed channel most often occurring between two loops of intestine or between the intestine and another structure, such as the bladder, vagina, or skin. Fistulas are much more common in Crohn's disease than in ulcerative colitis.

Flare-up
    See exacerbation.

Folic Acid
    One of the vitamins responsible for maintaining adequate production of red blood cells by bone marrow. A deficiency of folic acid may occur in IBD patients, particularly in those taking sulfasalazine. Oral supplements of folic acid are often provided to those with folic acid deficiency.

Fulminant
    Developing suddenly and severely.

Gastroenterologist
    A physician specializing in the diagnosis and treatment of patients with gastrointestinal diseases.

Granulomas
    Microscopic abnormalities within the intestinal wall detectable only by biopsy; characteristic of Crohn's disease but not of ulcerative colitis.

Gut
    Another word for the intestine or bowel.

Hemorrhoids
    Dilated, often painful veins susceptible to bleeding within the lower rectum and anus, sometimes seen as a complication in patients with IBD.

Hyperalimentation
    See parenteral nutrition.

Ileoanal anastomosis
    A newer operation for ulcerative colitis. After removal of the large intestine (colectomy), a pouch is made from the lower region of the small intestine (ileum). This pouch is attached directly to the anal opening. Stools are then evacuated through the anus in a normal manner. Also known as the ileoanal pull-through.

Ileostomy
    The diversion of fecal waste to a surgically created attachment of the ileum to the abdominal wall. Waste collects in a bag or appliance attached to the skin by special adhesive.

Immunology
The study of the immune response to disease in humans and animals.

Incontinence
The inability to retain feces, resulting in leakage to undergarments. In IBD, this usually occurs as a result of rectal inflammation.

Inflammation
A condition characterized by pain, heat, redness, and swelling.

Irritable Bowel Syndrome (IBS)
Abnormal contractions of the small and large intestine that often cause diarrhea and abdominal pain. IBS is often mistakenly called spastic colitis, although IBS is not associated with actual injury (inflammation) of the intestine and, therefore, has no relationship to IBD.

Laxative
A remedy that moves the bowels slightly without pain or violent action.

Microbiology
The science concerned with microscopic and ultramicroscopic organisms.

MRI
Magnetic resonance imaging, a radiologic procedure that makes use of a superconducting magnet, which then vibrates hydrogen molecules within the body and provides images of a particular part of the body.

Mucus
A clear or whitish jelly-like substance produced by the intestine which may be found in the stool.

Nasogastric Tube
A thin, flexible tube passed through the nose into the stomach. Also known as an NG tube. This tube can be used to withdraw fluid and air that may collect in the stomach when the bowel is obstructed or following intestinal surgery. It can also be used to deliver a liquid diet directly into the stomach and thereby eliminate the need for chewing and swallowing.

Nuclear scan
A test done by a radiologist in which a material is injected intravenously in order to "illuminate" a particular organ or organs. In IBD,

red cell scans are sometimes used to look for sources of bleeding. White cell scans are used to look for abscess pockets.

Obstruction
A blockage of the small or large intestine preventing the normal passage of intestinal contents. In Crohn's disease, obstruction may be caused by narrowing (stricture) or spasms of the intestine. Signs of obstruction are vomiting, abdominal pain, and distention of the abdomen.

Occult blood
Blood invisible to the naked eye which is found in stool. It is often an indication of intestinal inflammation or of relapsed IBD. Occult blood is ordinarily detected in laboratory tests.

Parenteral nutrition
An effort to provide some or all of the body's nutritional needs intravenously through a special intravenous (IV) line termed a catheter. Total parenteral nutrition (TPN) is used to provide adequate nutrition to severely ill or malnourished IBD patients. It is also sometimes used to provide bowel rest when medications are not working satisfactorily, or to prepare poorly nourished patients for surgery.

Perforation
An abnormal hole in the intestinal wall which causes intestinal contents to spill into the normally sterile abdominal cavity, leading to inflammation (peritonitis) or abscess formation.

Perianal
An area around the anal opening which may become inflamed and irritated in persons with IBD, especially Crohn's disease.

Proctocolectomy
Surgical removal of the entire colon and rectum.

Pyoderma gangrenosum
A type of skin sore that sometimes occurs on the extremities of persons with ulcerative colitis or Crohn's disease.

Remission
A diminishing or cessation of symptoms or disease activity.

Resection
Surgical removal of a diseased portion of intestine. Reattachment of the two ends of healthy bowel is called anastomosis.

Sclerosing cholangitis
A rare type of liver disease that may occur in association with IBD. It is more common in adults than in children.

Sigmoidoscopy
A test in which a lighted tube is passed through the anus and the sigmoid colon. Biopsies may be taken through the sigmoidoscope. Sedation is sometimes needed for patient comfort during the procedure.

Stricture
A narrowed area of intestine caused by inflammation or scar tissue.

Suppository
A semisolid medical substance, commonly shaped like a cylinder or cone, for insertion into the rectum. Suppositories often serve as a vehicle for topical medicines intended to reduce inflammations.

Tenesmus
The persistent urge to empty the bowel or bladder, with involuntary, ineffectual straining efforts.

Toxic megacolon
A rare but sudden and extreme widening of the colon, more common in ulcerative colitis than Crohn's disease. A serious condition, which may lead to severe illness or perforation, sometimes necessitating colectomy.

Tube Feeding
Delivery of a liquid diet by a tube, usually passed through the nose into the stomach or small intestine.

Ultrasound examination
A test employing sound waves (sonar) performed by a radiologist to identify internal body structures. In a person with IBD, an abdominal ultrasound exam might be used to look for an abscess.

Upper endoscopy
Endoscopic examination of the upper gastrointestinal tract with a lighted tube to look for abnormalities of the stomach and upper small intestine in particular. Sedation is often given for comfort during the procedure.

Upper GI series
An x-ray examination of the esophagus, stomach, and upper small

intestine (duodenum). X-rays are taken after liquid barium is swallowed on an empty stomach. The test can be extended to permit the illumination of the entire small intestine, including the ileum. The x-ray is then known as an upper GI series with small bowel follow-through.

Uveitis

A complication of IBD affecting the eyes, causing redness and discomfort and requiring treatment by an ophthalmologist.

CHILDREN'S LEGACY SCROLL OF HONOR

**Dedicated to the Advancement of Research and Therapy
In Inflammatory Bowel Disease**

A
Adina M. Aaron
Fred L. Aaron
Greg Aarons
Jacob Agris
Laurel Ann Agris
Adi Reicher Alouf
Mark Alpert
Nicol Alpert
Scott Alpert
Deborah Miller Ambroze
Wayne L. Ambroze, Jr. , M.D.
Jude Anheluk
Andrea Arno
Frances B. Austell
Jane Austin

B
Judith Lauter Baer
Katherine Balio
Ahmie, Sara, Brian, & Melissa Baum
Christine Baum
Evelyn & Jack Bayer
Martin & Kathleen Beirne
Mr. & Mrs. Robert Bekoff
Daniela Bell
Mr. & Mrs. Leo Benatar
Mr. & Mrs. Morris L. Benatar
Michael Berger, M.D.
Irvin Berman
Joan B. Berman
Dana M. Bernstein
Edward M. Bernstein
Drew Tyler Birch

Erica Lee Birch
Jessica Lynn Birch
Flora Bishop
Kristine Bishop
Jean & Edward Biskind
H.E. "Bud" Blaksley
Marsha, Stephen, Cheryl, & Lisa Blank
Lillian & Richard Blucher
Brian Bluestein
Dr. Jason & Pearlena Bodzin
Mr. & Mrs. Michael J. Boling
Dorothy L. Bosken
Conner and Chase Boyle
Sanford Cunningham Bradshaw
Joshua Bross
Mark Brottman
Mr. & Mrs. Hal Browning
Bobbi Burke
Kevin Burge
Chase Byrd

C
Debbie J. Callan
Richard O. & Dorothy M. Campbell
Carla S. Caputo
Caroline, Francis, Hassie & Bailey
Karen Chase
Kristy Cocuzzo
Mr. & Mrs. John L. Cohn
Leon & Toby Cooperman
Gertrude F. Coords

D
Lawrence C. Dailey
Roberta J. Dailey
Benjamin & Frances David
Leon Davis
Mr. & Mrs. George C. Denby
Lisa Ditchek-Levenson, Psy.D.
Kimberly Oteri Dollard

Stuart & Leslie Dubin

E
Justin David Einstein
Valerie Jaye Elston
Deena J. Esensten
Ruth & Maury Ettleson
Mark E. Evans

F
Howard Fensterman
Lori Fensterman
Dr. & Mrs. George Ferry
Arnold & Sheila Fieldman
Warren Finkelstein, M.D
Aron Fisch
Jerry Fisher
Joan Fisher
Bruce Flack
Shirley & Harvey Flomenhoft
Eleanore Foonberg
Harold Foonberg
Barbara Foster
Mara C. Fribush
Dale B. Fuller
Lynne N. Fuller

G
Raymond & Shirley Galant
Joan Geduld
Irwin Geduld
Mr. & Mrs. John Gee
Dr. & Mrs. Maxwell Gelfand
Annette Lynn Michaelson Giarla
Allison Beth Glazer
Joshua Alan Glazer
Dorey Glen
Lynn Goodman
Gene & Kaitlin Joy Gottfried
Rebecca Gould

Barbara & Bernard Green
Robert & Cathy Greenly

H
Steven & June Haber
Mr. & Mrs. Michel T. Halbouty
Mrs. Chester Hamilton
Rebekah Ruth Hampton
Robert Hardi, M.D.
The Hartstein Family
Barbara & Louis Henkind
Henry M. Hermann
Edward Courtland Hill
Patrick William Hill
Nancy Jones Homeyer
Jacob Hopper
Lindsay Hopper
Michael Horan
Mr. & Mrs. Stephen Horan
Megan Huard
Eleanor Joanna Huffman

I
The Inner Circle, Inc.

J
Elijah David Jackson
Robin Jacobs
Douglas Johnson
Sonya L. Johnson

K
Alison Leigh Kacyra
David Aaron Kahn
Mario D. Kamionowski, M.D.
Nicole, Alissa, Oren, & Gauriele Kantor
Jill & Myron Kaplan
David Karas
Kara Karas
Holly Katz

Howard C. Katz
Morton L. Katz, Ph.D
Thomas J. Kelly, M.D.
Hannah Eve Kerman
Thomas Kiel-Fie
Hunter Kiely
Lindsay Kiely
Mr. & Mrs. Harold Kittay
Mita Klein
Jason Kling
Laurie Koh
Linda L. Konrad
Judith Naomi Kops
Jason M. Korkin
Randi M. Korobelnik
Bernard J. Kost
J. Hunt Kost
Dr. & Mrs. M. Krasman
Howard S. Kroop, M.D.
Ross David Kulberg

L
Joan & Edwin Lasner
William Pat Leake
Dr. & Mrs. Peter B. Leff
Don & Mary Jo Lenauer
Julia Lesley
Fred. A Levin, M. D.
Clarie Levine
Felice Levine
Debra Galant Levinson
Fay J. Lindner Foundation
Danielle Linehan
Jalayna Ann Linnebur
Scott Liptzin
Jeremy Lowenstein

M
Michael I. Margolis
Mr. & Mrs. I. W. Marks

Elizabeth Marmon
Rusty A. McIntosh
Kevin McNicholas
C. Brian Melonakos
Allie Miller
Kevin Miller
Charles V. Moran
Jim & Jan Moran
Lorene G. Moran
Mr. & Mrs. Michael B. Moran
Courtney Alexa Moskovitz
Jayne Rosenwald Myers
John M. & Tara J. Myers, M. D.

N
The Robert Naponic Family

O
Guy R. Orangio, M.D.
Loulou Anne Orenstein

P
Michael A. Palladino
Mr. & Mrs. Gerald L. Parsky
John & Denise Peck
Rachel Pender
Stuart Pflaum
Brieanne Phillips
Carole A. Pinkett
Brian Piper
Jeffrey Piscopo
Sheila Brown Piscopo
Christopher Troy Price
John Vernon Price
Procter & Gamble Pharmaceuticals

R
Reach Out for Youth with
   Ileitis and Colitis, Inc.
Laura Reeder

Cecily Wenzel Reichard
Jeffrey C. Rice
Lisa Richardson
Michelle Renee Rifkin
Laura Anne Robbin
Carol & Skip Roberts
Juan Carlos Artaza Roca
Ophelia A. Roca
Richard & Kim Rolland
Rebecca Rose
Cynthia Ann Rosen
Ms. Sunny Rosen
Sylvia Catherine Rosenwald
Fred C. Rothstein, M. D.
Melvin & Jean Ruben

S
John S. Sabel, M.D.
David Sales, M.D., Ph.D.
Carli L. Salzberg
Lindsay E. Salzberg
Matthew Sanderson
Audrey & Herb Saperstein
Megan Saphir
Aaron Sapiro
Nicole Sapiro
Anne L Saris, M. D.
Scott Savage
Mr. & Mrs. Bennett M. Schlenger
Benjamin Schlossmann
Schnader, Harrison, Segal & Lewis
Sid & Suzanne Schneider
Dr. & Mrs. Matthew Schwartz
Foster J. Scott, Jr.
Kelly Ann Scott
Emily Elizabeth Seligmann
Matthew Filer Seligmann
Sam Allen Seligmann
Matthew C. Serkes & Family
Jessica Shacklett

Mickey & Al Shankman
Rachel Shankman
Sid & Suzanne Shneider
Dr. & Mrs. Matthew Shwartz
Jaimi Silk
Barry Silverman
Daren Simkin
Megan Elizabeth Smith
Robin & Steven Smith
Thomas H. Smith, Jr.
Mr. & Mrs. Rollin J. Soskin
P. Bruce Spain
Susan Spellman
Erica Paige Sperling
Marion & Don Stadler
Joshua Robert Stein
Melanie Robyn Stein
Tina & Gary Steinbeck
Michael Isaac Steingold
Donna B. Stewart
Bud & Rose Strauss
Mr. & Mrs. Michael Strauss
William & Arlene Strauss
Dr. & Mrs. Steven J. Stryker
Emily Swanson

T
Dr. & Mrs. Stephan R. Targan & Family
Talbot Scott Taylor
Jane Louden Thomas
Scott Thompson
Eric & Elspeth Thomson

V
Gary & Lynette Vajda
Marian Van Derlaske

W
Alison, Bob & Elizabeth Wachstein
Mr. & Mrs. J. Virgil Waggoner

Phyllis Wayne
Bernard & Frances Willig
Brooke Taylor Willis
Mr. & Mrs. Michael T. Willis
Alice & Larry Wolf
Adam Wolfert
Mark & Brian Wolly

Z
The Zarrow Families
David C. Zweig

In Honor of Cathy Brooks, Our Sister

In Honor of Rosalyn C. Richman

In Memory of Cheryl Ryave Radov

MasterMedia Limited

To order copies of *Managing Your Child's Crohn's Disease or Ulcerative Colitis* ($21.95), send a check for the price of each book ordered plus $2 postage and handling for the first book and $1 for each additional copy to:

MasterMedia Limited
17 East 89th Street
New York, NY 10128
(212) 546-7650
(800) 334-8232
(212) 546-7638 (fax)
(Please use MasterCard or VISA on phone orders)

An Invitation

If you found this book helpful and want to receive a MasterMedia book catalog or a newsletter that contains a list of MasterMedia's inspirational books that carry the Heritage Imprint, write or fax to the above address or phone number.

MasterMedia is the only company to combine publishing with a full-service speakers' bureau.

MasterMedia books and speakers cover today's important issues— from family values to health topics and business ethics.

For information and a complete list of speakers, call (800) 453-2887 or fax (908) 359-1647.

OTHER MASTERMEDIA BOOKS

To order additional copies of any MasterMedia book, send a check for the price of the book plus $2.00 postage and handling for the first book, $1.00 for each additional book to:

MasterMedia Limited
17 East 89th Street
New York, NY 10128
(212) 546-7650
(800) 334-8232
(212) 546-7638 (fax)
(Please use MasterCard or VISA on phone orders)

AGING PARENTS AND YOU: A Complete Handbook to Help You Help Your Elders Maintain a Healthy, Productive and Independent Life, by Eugenia Anderson-Ellis, is a complete guide to providing care to aging relatives. It gives practical advice and resources to adults who are helping their elders lead productive and independent lives. Revised and updated. ($9.95 paper)

BALANCING ACTS! Juggling Love, Work, Family, and Recreation, by Susan Schiffer Stautberg and Marcia L. Worthing, provides strategies to achieve a balanced life by reordering priorities and setting realistic goals. ($12.95 paper)

BEATING THE AGE GAME: Redefining Retirement, by Jack and Phoebe Ballard, debunks the myth that retirement means sitting out the rest of the game. The years between 55 and 80 can be your best, say the authors, who provide ample examples of people successfully using retirement to reinvent their lives. ($12.95 paper)

THE BIG APPLE BUSINESS AND PLEASURE GUIDE: 501 Ways to Work Smarter, Play Harder, and Live Better in New York City, by Muriel Siebert and Susan Kleinman, offers visitors and New Yorkers alike advice on how to do business in the city and enjoy its attractions. ($9.95 paper)

BREATHING SPACE: Living and Working at a Comfortable Pace in a Sped-Up Society, by Jeff Davidson, helps readers to handle information and activity overload and gain greater control over their lives. ($10.95 paper)

CARVING WOOD AND STONE, by Arnold Prince, is an illustrated step-by-step handbook demonstrating all you need to hone your wood and carving skills. ($11.95 paper)

THE COLLEGE COOKBOOK II, for Students by Students, by Nancy Levicki, is a handy volume of recipes culled from college students across the U.S. ($11.95)

THE CONFIDENCE FACTOR: How Self-Esteem Can Change Your Life, by Dr. Judith Briles, is based on a nationwide survey of six thousand men and women. Briles explores why women so often feel a lack of self-confidence and have a poor opinion of themselves. She offers step-by-step advice on becoming the person you want to be. ($9.95 paper, $18.95 cloth)

CUPID, COUPLES & CONTRACTS: A Guide to Living Together, Prenuptial Agreements, and Divorce, by Lester Wallman, with Sharon McDonnell, is an insightful, consumer-oriented handbook that provides a comprehensive overview of family law, including prenuptial agreements, alimony and fathers' rights ($12.95 paper)

THE DOLLARS AND SENSE OF DIVORCE: The Financial Guide for Women, by Dr. Judith Briles, is the first book to combine the legal hurdles by planning finances before, during and after divorce. ($10.95 paper)

FINANCIAL SAVVY FOR WOMEN: A Money Book for Women of All Ages, by Dr. Judith Briles, divides a woman's monetary lifespan into six phases, discusses specific issues to be addressed at each stage and demonstrates how to create a sound money plan. ($15.00 paper)

FLIGHT PLAN FOR LIVING: The Art of Self-Encouragement, by Patrick O'Dooley, is a guide organized like a pilot's checklist, to ensure you'll by flying "clear to the top" throughout your life. ($17.95 cloth)

HOT HEALTH-CARE CAREERS, by Margaret McNally and Phyllis Schneider, offers readers what they need to know about training for and getting jobs in a rewarding field where professionals are always in demand. ($10.95 paper)

HOW TO GET WHAT YOU WANT FROM ALMOST ANYBODY, by T. Scott Gross, shows how to get great service, negotiate better prices and always get what you pay for. ($9.95 paper)

KIDS WHO MAKE A DIFFERENCE, by Joyce Roché and Marie Rodriguez, is an inspiring document on how today's toughest challenges are being met by teenagers and kids, whose courage and creativity enables them to find practical solutions! ($8.95 paper, with photos)

LEADING YOUR POSITIVELY OUTRAGEOUS SERVICE TEAM, by T. Scott Gross, forgoes theory in favor of a hands-on approach. Gross provides a step-by-step formula for developing self-managing service teams that put the customer first. ($12.95 paper)

LIFE'S THIRD ACT: Taking Control of Your Mature Years, by Patricia Burnham, Ph.D., is a perceptive handbook for everyone who recognizes that planning is the key to enjoying your mature years. ($10.95 paper, $18.95 cloth)

LIFETIME EMPLOYABILITY: How to Become Indispensable, by Carole Hyatt is both a guide through the mysteries of the business universe brought down to earth and a handbook to help you evaluate your attitudes, your skills, and your goals. Through expert advice and interviews of nearly 200 men and women whose lives have changed because their jobs or goals shifted, *Lifetime Employability* is designed to increase your staying power in today's down-sized economy. ($12.95 paper)

LISTEN TO WIN: A Guide to Effective Listening, by Curt Bechler, Ph.D., and Richard Weaver, Ph.D., is a powerful, people-oriented book that will help you learn to live with others, connect with them and get the best from them. ($18.95 cloth)

THE LIVING HEART BRAND NAME SHOPPER'S GUIDE, by Michael F. DeBakey, M.D., Antonio M. Gotto, Jr., M.D., Lynne W. Scott, M.A., R.D./L.D., and John P. Foreyt, Ph.D., lists brand-name supermarket products that are low in fat, saturated fatty acids, and cholesterol. ($12.50 paper)

THE LIVING HEART GUIDE TO EATING OUT, by Michael F. DeBakey, M.D., Antonio M. Gotto, Jr., M.D., and Lynne W. Scott, M.A., R.D./L.D., is an essential handbook for people who want to maintain a health-conscious diet when dining in all types of restaurants. ($9.95 paper)

MAKING YOUR DREAMS COME TRUE NOW!, by Marcia Wieder, introduces an easy, unique, and practical technique for defining, pursuing, and realizing your career and life interests. Filled with stories of real people and helpful exercises, plus a personal workbook. (Revised and updated. $10.95 paper)

MANAGING IT ALL: Time-Saving Ideas for Career, Family, Relationships, and Self, by Beverly Benz Treuille and Susan Schiffer Stautberg, is written for women who are juggling careers and families. More than 200 career women (ranging from a TV anchorwoman to an investment baker) were interviewed. The book contains many humorous anecdotes on saving time and improving the quality of life for self and family. ($9.95 paper)

MANAGING YOUR CHILD'S DIABETES, by Robert Wood Johnson IV, Sale Johnson, Casey Johnson, and Susan Kleinman, brings help to families trying to understand diabetes and control its effects. ($10.95 paper)

MANAGING YOUR PSORIASIS, by Nicholas J. Lowe, M.D., is an innovative manual that couples scientific research and encouraging support, with an emphasis on how patients can take charge of their health. ($10.95 paper, $17.95 cloth)

MANN FOR ALL SEASONS: Wit and Wisdom from The Washington Post's Judy Mann, shows the columnist at her best as she writes about women, families and the impact and politics of the women's revolution. ($9.95 paper, $19.95 cloth)

MEMORY: Remembering and Forgetting in Everyday Life, by Dr. Barry Gordon, explains the difference between a real memory impairment and the normal absent-mindedness that affects us all. ($25.00 cloth)

MIND YOUR OWN BUSINESS: And Keep It in the Family, by Marcy Syms, CEO of Syms Corp., is an effective guide for any organization facing the toughest step in managing a family business—making the transition to the new generation. ($12.95 paper, $18.95 cloth)

OFFICE BIOLOGY: Why Tuesday Is the Most Productive Day and Other Relevant Facts for Survival in the Workplace, by Edith Weiner and Arnold Brown, teaches how in the '90s and beyond we will be expected to work smarter, take better control of our health, adapt to advancing technology, and improve our lives in ways that are not too costly or resource-intensive. ($12.95 paper, $21.95 cloth)

ON TARGET: Enhance Your Life and Advance Your Career, by Jeri Sedlar and Rick Miners, is a neatly woven tapestry of insights on career and life issues gathered from audiences across the country. This feedback has been crystallized into a highly readable guide for exploring what you want. ($11.95 paper)

PAIN RELIEF: How to Say No to Acute, Chronic, and Cancer Pain!, by Dr. Jane Cowles, offers a step-by-step plan for assessing pain and communicating it to your doctor, and explains the importance of having a pain plan before undergoing any medical or surgical treatment; includes "The Pain Patient's Bill of Rights," and a reusable pain assessment chart. ($14.95 paper, 22.95 cloth)

POSITIVELY OUTRAGEOUS SERVICE: New and Easy Ways to Win Customers for Life, by T. Scott Gross, identifies what '90s consumers really want and how business can develop effective marketing strategies to answer those needs. ($14.95 paper)

THE PREGNANCY AND MOTHERHOOD DIARY: Planning the First Year of Your Second Career, by Susan Schiffer Stautberg, is the first and only undated appointment diary that shows how to manage pregnancy and career. ($12.95, spiral bound)

ROSEY GRIER'S ALL-AMERICAN HEROES: Multicultural Success Stories, by Roosevelt "Rosey" Grier, is a candid collection of profiles of prominent African-Americans, Latins, Asians and Native Americans who reveal how they achieved public acclaim and personal success. ($9.95 paper, with photos)

A SEAT AT THE TABLE: An Insider's Guide for America's New Women Leaders, by Patricia Harrison. A must-read guide that offers practical advice for women who want to serve on boards of directors, play key roles in politics and community affairs or become policy makers in public or private sectors. ($19.95 cloth)

SELLING YOURSELF: Be the Competent, Confident Person You Really Are!, by Kathy Thebo, Joyce Newman and Diana Lynn. The ability to express yourself effectively and to project a confident image is essential in today's fast-paced world where professional and personal lines frequently cross. ($12.95 paper)

SHOCKWAVES. The Global Impact of Sexual Harassment, by Susan L. Webb, examines the problem of sexual harassment today in every kind of workplace around the world. Well-researched, this manual provides the most recent information available, including legal changes in progress. ($11.95 paper, $19.95 cloth)

SOMEONE ELSE'S SON, by Alan Winter, explores the parent-child bond in a contemporary novel of lost identities, family secrets and relationships gone awry. Eighteen years after bringing their first son home from the hospital, Tish and Brad Hunter discover they are not his biological parents. ($18.95 cloth)

STEP FORWARD: Sexual Harassment in the Workplace, What You Need to Know, by Susan L. Webb, presents the facts for identifying the telltale signs of sexual harassment on the job, and how to deal with it. ($9.95 paper)

THE STEPPARENT CHALLENGE: A Primer for Making it Work, by Stephen Williams, Ph.D., offers insight into the many aspects of step relationships—from financial issues to lifestyle changes to differences in race and or religion that affect the whole family. ($13.95 paper)

STRAIGHT TALK ON WOMEN'S HEALTH: How to Get the Health Care You Deserve, by Janice Teal, Ph.D., and Phyllis Schneider, is destined to become a health-care "bible." Devoid of confusing medical jargon, it offers a wealth of resources, including contact lists of health lines and women's medical centers. ($14.95 paper)

TEAMBUILT: Making Teamwork Work, by Mark Sanborn, teaches business how to increase productivity, without increasing resources or expenses, by building teamwork among employees. ($12.95 paper, $19.95 cloth)

A TEEN'S GUIDE TO BUSINESS: The Secrets to a Successful Enterprise, by Linda Menzies, Oren Jenkins, and Rick Fisher, provides solid information about starting your own business or working for one. ($7.95 paper)

WHAT KIDS LIKE TO DO, by Edward Stautberg, Gail Wubbenhorst, Ativa Easterling, and Phyllis Schneider, is a handy guide for parents, grandparents and sitters. Written by kids, this is an easy-to-read, generously illustrated primer for teaching families how to make every day more fun. ($7.95 paper).

WHEN THE WRONG THING IS RIGHT: How to Overcome Conventional Wisdom, Popular Opinion and All the Lies Your Parents Told You, by Sylvia Bigelson, Ed.S., and Virginia McCullough, addresses issues such as marriage, relationships, parents and siblings, divorce, sex, money and careers, and encourages readers to break free from the pressures of common wisdom and to trust their own choices. ($9.95 paper)

WHY MEN MARRY: Insights from Marrying Men, by A. T. Langford, interviews 64 men, revealing their views on marriage. These men describe what scares them about women, how potential partners are tested and how it feels to be a "marriage object." ($18.95 cloth)

A WOMAN'S PLACE IS EVERYWHERE: Inspiration Profiles of Female Leaders Who Are Expanding the Roles of American Women, by Lindsey Johnson and Jackie Joyner-Kersee, profiles 30 women whose personal and professional achievements are helping to shape and expand our ideas of what's possible for humankind. ($9.95 paper)

THE WORKING MOM ON THE RUN MANUAL: by Debbie Nigro, is a humorous, practical guide for working parents, particularly single, working moms. Offers insights about careers, disciplining the kids, coping with husbands who won't do housework, running a home-based business and keeping track of just about everything every day. ($9.95 paper)

YOUR VISION: All About Modern Eye Care, by Warren D. Cross Jr., M.D., and Lawrence Lynn, Ph.D., reveals astounding research discoveries in an entertaining and informative handbook written with the patient in mind. ($13.95 paper)

WORLD RIDE: Going the Extra Mile Against Cancer, by Richard Drorbaugh, is a fast-paced, high-spirited, humorous and passionate narrative that dramatizes the mission—a 32-country bike tour—the author and his two teammates undertook to bring global attention to a universal disease. ($11.95 paper)

THE HERITAGE IMPRINT OF INSPIRATIONAL BOOKS

MasterMedia's Heritage Imprint books speak of courage, integrity and bouncing back from defeat. For the millions of Americans seeking greater purpose and meaning in their lives in difficult times, here are volumes of inspiration, solace and spiritual support.

The Heritage Imprint books are supported by MasterMedia's full-service speakers' bureau, authors' media and lecture tours, syndicated radio interviews, national and co-op advertising and publicity.

AMERICAN HEROES: Their Lives, Their Values, Their Beliefs, by Dr. Robert B. Pamplin, Jr., with Gary K. Eisler, demonstrates that courage, integrity, compassion, the qualities of the hero, still live in American men and women today—even in a world that is filled with disillusionment. Share their stories of outstanding achievements, and discover the values that guide their lives as revealed in a pioneering coast-to-coast survey. ($18.95 cloth)

THE ETHICAL EDGE: Tales of Organizations That Have Faced Moral Crises, by Dawn-Marie Driscoll, W. Michael Hoffman, Edward S. Petry, associated with The Center for Business Ethics at Bentley College, links the current search for meaning and values in life with stories of corporate turnarounds. Read about organizations that have recovered from moral crises and the tough lessons they've learned and the ethical structures they've put in place to ensure a solid future. ($24.95 cloth)

HERITAGE: The Making of the American Family, by Robert B. Pamplin, Jr., Gary K. Eisler, Jeff Sengstack and John Domini, mixes history and philosophy in a biographical saga of the Pamplins' phenomenal ascent to wealth and the creation of one of the largest private fortunes in the U.S. ($24.95 cloth)

JOURNEY TOWARD FORGIVENESS: Finding Your Way Home, by BettyClare Moffatt, is a delightfully positive inspirational self-help book that provides spiritual guidelines to forgiveness, meditation, prayer, action, healing and change. ($11.95 paper)

PRELUDE TO SURRENDER: The Pamplin Family and the Siege of Petersburg, by Robert B. Pamplin, Jr., with Gary K. Eisler, Jeff Sengstack and John Domini, is an engaging account of how the author's ancestral home was taken over by the Confederacy for use as a hospital and as a defensive position. It is now the Pamplin Park Civil War Site. ($10.95 paper)

RESILIENCY: How to Bounce Back Faster, Stronger, Smarter, by Tessa Albert Warschaw, Ph.D., and Dee Barlow, Ph.D., is packed with practical techniques and insights on solving old problems in new ways.

The book also shows readers how to become more resilient in their personal and professional lives and teaches the skills for bouncing back from everyday stresses to surviving disastrous multiple losses. You will learn to enthusiastically embrace life. ($21.95 cloth)

You Choose Stories: Scooby-Doo
is published by Stone Arch Books,
A Capstone Imprint
1710 Roe Crest Drive
North Mankato, Minnesota 56003
www.capstonepub.com

CAPS30180

Cataloging-in-Publication Data is available on the
Library of Congress website.
ISBN: 978-1-4342-6404-6 [Library Hardcover]
ISBN: 978-1-4342-7925-5 [Paperback]

Summary: Scooby-Doo and the gang need your
help solving the secret of the sea creature
in this You Choose mystery!

Printed in the United States of America in Stevens Point, Wisconsin.
092013   007765WZS14

SCOOBY-DOO!

THE SECRET OF THE SEA CREATURE

written by
Laurie S. Sutton

illustrated by
Scott Neely

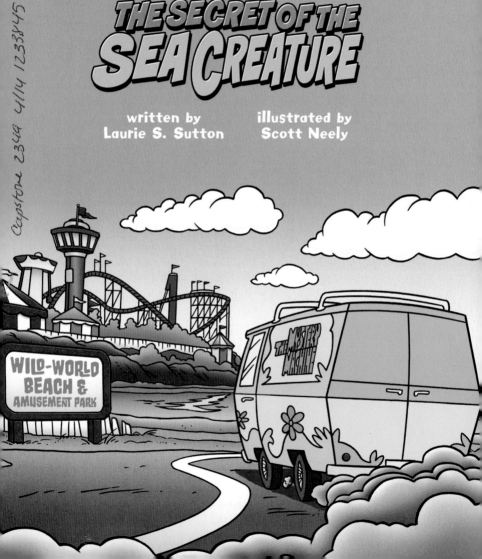

WILD-WORLD
BEACH &
AMUSEMENT PARK

THE MYSTERY INC. GANG!

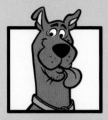

SCOOBY-DOO

SKILLS: Loyal; super snout
BIO: This happy-go-lucky hound avoids scary situations at all costs, but he'll do anything for a Scooby Snack!

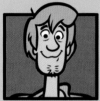

SHAGGY ROGERS

SKILLS: Lucky; healthy appetite
BIO: This laid-back dude would rather look for grub than search for clues, but he usually finds both!

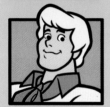

FRED JONES, JR.

SKILLS: Athletic; charming
BIO: The leader and oldest member of the gang. He's a good sport—and good at them, too!

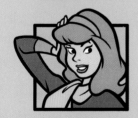

DAPHNE BLAKE

SKILLS: Brains; beauty
BIO: As a sixteen-year-old fashion queen, Daphne solves her mysteries in style.

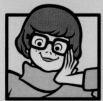

VELMA DINKLEY

SKILLS: Clever; highly intelligent
BIO: Although she's the youngest member of Mystery Inc., Velma's an old pro at catching crooks.

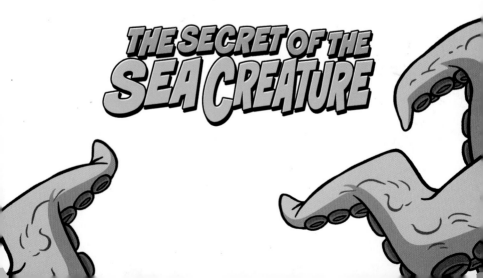

← YOU CHOOSE →

SCOOBY-DOO!

™

A sea creature is on the loose at **Wild-World Beach!** Only **YOU** can help Scooby-Doo and the Mystery Inc. gang solve this maritime mystery.

Follow the directions at the bottom of each page. The choices **YOU** make will change the outcome of the story. After you finish one path, go back and read the others for more Scooby-Doo adventures!

YOU CHOOSE the path to solve...

THE SECRET OF THE SEA CREATURE

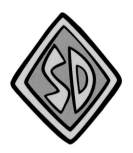

On a hot, steamy day, the Mystery Machine zooms down the highway. Fred Jones, Jr. is at the wheel of the lime-green van. He's the leader of Mystery Inc., a gang of teenage crime solvers, but today is all about summer fun.

"What a great day for a drive to the beach!" says Daphne from the passenger seat.

"Like, are we there yet?" Shaggy moans.

"Ryeah, are we rhere yet?" Scooby-Doo whimpers from the back seat. "Ri'm hungry!"

"You guys are always hungry," Velma points out, pushing her glasses up her nose. "You don't have stomachs. You two have bottomless pits!"

Turn the page.

"Aw, Velma," Shaggy replies. "Like, we just can't wait to taste those famous Wild-World Beach hot dogs. Right, boy?"

"Ryeah! Rummy!" says Scooby, licking his lips. Drool drips from the dog's long, wagging tongue.

"Well, you can eat all the hot dogs you want," Velma says. "I'm more interested in the rare shells." She pulls out a book about seashells.

"Yuck! I don't like snails," Shaggy exclaims.

"Not snails—shells!" Velma says. "Wild-World Beach is home to the *Conus beautificus*, also known as the Jewel of the Sea." She opens her book to a picture of the rainbow-colored shell.

"Yeah, and it's also a great place to snorkel," Fred adds, glancing back at them in the rearview mirror. "That's what I'm going to do!"

"I didn't know you liked to snorkel, Fred," says Daphne.

"Oh, sure," Fred replies with a proud grin. "I'm an all-round sports-type dude."

"What are you going to do at Wild-World, Daphne?" Velma asks.

"I'm going hunting," Daphne replies.

"WHAT?!" the gang shouts together. Fred is so surprised he nearly drives off the road.

"Like, lions, tigers, and bears, and stuff?" Shaggy says with a loud gulp.

"Rhose poor rittle ranimals!" Scooby-Doo whimpers, covering his eyes with a paw.

Daphne shows them a flashy magazine, which is filled with dozens of photographs of celebrities and other famous people on the cover. "Not animal hunting, silly. Celebrity hunting!" she explains. "I read that movie stars like to go to this beach. Maybe I can meet one."

"Rhew!" exclaims Scooby, relieved.

Turn the page.

Just then, the Mystery Machine drives past a road sign that points to the exit for Wild-World Beach and Amusement Park.

"We're here!" Shaggy says. "I can almost smell those foot-long hot dogs with all the fixings."

"Rippeee!" Scooby-Doo agrees. His snout twitches wildly. "I smell rhem right now!"

Scooby's legs spin like pinwheels as he gets ready to run. Fred barely has enough time to drive the van onto the exit before Shaggy and Scooby-Doo are out the door and down the road.

"I guess we'll meet them there," says Velma.

Fred parks the Mystery Machine not far from the beach. The gang climbs out of the van and looks around. The beach is jam-packed with people. Kids are with their moms and dads. A group plays volleyball. Friends toss a football. Everyone is having fun.

They can see the rides in the amusement park and the kite surfers on the water. They don't see Shaggy or Scooby-Doo, but that doesn't worry them. Those two chowhounds are easy to find— just look for a food stand!

"I'm off to search for shells," Velma says.

"And I'm going kitesurfing," adds Daphne.

The two girls head toward the beach.

"Okay, let's split up for now," Fred suggests, jogging toward the surf.

To follow Velma, turn to page 12.

To follow Shaggy & Scooby, turn to page 13.

To follow Daphne, turn to page 14.

To follow Fred, turn to page 16.

Leaving the Mystery Inc. gang, Velma walks along the beach, searching for the Jewel of the Sea. With her head down, she concentrates on finding one of the rare shells. But she doesn't see anything except sand. "Not many shells on the beach today," she says with a heavy sigh.

Suddenly, Velma hears shouting. *Did someone say "shark"?* she wonders.

Then, a nearby lifeguard warns people to get out of the water. *WEEEEEE!* He blows his whistle urgently. Velma looks up from her seashell search and sees people running from the beach.

A huge creature bursts up out of the surf like a powerful geyser. Velma quickly realizes that it's not a shark. It's much bigger and much more dangerous. It's a sea monster!

If Velma decides to take a closer look, turn to page 18.
If Velma waits on the beach for help, turn to page 63.

Away from the gang, Scooby-Doo and his best pal, Shaggy, quickly gulp down Wild-World Beach's famous hot dogs.

"It's dog-eat-dog, if you know what I mean, Scoob!" says Shaggy, chuckling.

"Ryeah!" Scooby agrees. "Ri never met a rog Ri didn't rike."

The friends lick their lips with big sloppy tongues. They don't need napkins. Every trace of ketchup, mustard, relish, onions, pickles, cheese, and chili is gone in a single swipe!

"Row about rotton candy?" Scooby suggests.

"Like, there's nothing better than spun sugar on a stick!" Shaggy says. "Let's go!"

Hurrying along the pier, they suddenly hear a burst of screaming!

If Shaggy & Scooby ignore the screams, turn to page 20.
If Shaggy & Scooby investigate the screams, turn to page 99.

After leaving the gang, Daphne rents a kiteboard and heads into the ocean. She zips across the surface of the water on her board as fast as the breeze can carry her. Daphne jumps and twists in the air, then lands with a splash.

SPA-LOOSH!

The bow-shaped sail above her head pulls Daphne parallel to the shore. She tries to look for celebrities on the beach as she surfs, but she's too busy controlling the kite.

"Maybe I should have stayed on land," Daphne says. "Besides, the sea spray is ruining my hair and makeup."

Suddenly, Daphne hears the lifeguard blow his whistle frantically. *What is he shouting?* she wonders, unable to hear him clearly.

"Why is everyone running off the beach?" she asks herself. "Am I missing something exciting?"

Daphne turns her kiteboard around to sail toward shore. That's when she sees what everyone is yelling about. A giant sea monster rises out of the water right in front of her!

"Jeepers!" Daphne exclaims.

The wind blows Daphne's kite straight toward the monster. She pulls on the lines and tries to turn her board.

Then, a strong gust catches the billowing sail and lifts Daphne high into the air. She is at the mercy of the sea breeze. The monster reaches out with its giant tentacles and tries to grab her.

"If this creepy creature catches me, I'm in real trouble!" Daphne says.

If Daphne lowers the kiteboard to the water, turn to page 24.
If Daphne lifts her kiteboard higher in the sky, turn to page 51.

After leaving the gang, Fred snorkels along an artificial reef. At first he floats on the surface and watches the fish swim among the plants and rocks. They are all the colors of the rainbow! Then Fred takes a deep breath and dives.

This is better than any aquarium! Fred thinks. *I could reach out and touch the fish—if they didn't swim so fast!*

Right then, something silvery catches his attention. It resembles a bright eel swimming through the water like a weightless snake. Fred has never seen anything like it, so he follows the unusual creature. It disappears into a crack in the reef.

Fred puts his face mask up to the crevice to look inside. A giant eyeball looks back!

Fred is so startled that he instinctively shouts under water. He exhales and all the breath leaves his lungs. Fred is forced to surface.

"What was that?" he says as he floats on top of the water. "I've got to investigate!"

Fred inhales an extra-deep breath this time. He dives back down to the reef. When he gets to the crack, he boldly peers inside. Nothing looks back at him.

Did I imagine it? Fred questions himself. *It seemed so real.*

Suddenly, something gigantic rises up out of the reef. It has silvery skin just like the eel and tentacles like a squid.

I didn't imagine anything. I saw a real sea monster! Fred realizes.

Turn to page 26.

Velma drops her stash of seashells and heads toward the water for a closer look. She isn't afraid of sea monsters. She and the Mystery Inc. gang are experts of the weird and mysterious.

"There's an explanation for everything!" Velma exclaims, creeping closer and closer to the strange, aquatic beast.

Suddenly, one of the monster's tentacles grabs Velma and lifts her high into the air. It shakes her so hard that her glasses almost fall off.

Velma is worried. "I can't see anything without my glasses!" she cries out.

The sea monster's tentacle has Velma in its grasp. **WHOOSH! WHOOSH!** It whips her in circles, around and around its head.

Moments later, Velma is right in front of its eyeball! She notices this is no ordinary eyeball. There's a man inside! He's in a control room.

"This monster is man-made," Velma realizes. "There *is* an explanation for everything!"

Velma wonders if she should try to escape from the mechanical monster's clutches. *If I struggle, the sea monster's controller might get even more upset,* she thinks.

She considers shouting for help instead. Maybe someone will save her in time.

If Velma tries to escape on her own, turn to page **29**.
If Velma shouts for help, turn to page **38**.

Shaggy and Scooby-Doo have their taste buds set on cotton candy. People are screaming, but the pals pay no attention. It's the sound of people having fun on the rides, right?

Suddenly, a mob thunders over Scooby and Shaggy. People are in a panic!

Whoa! What's the rush? Shaggy wonders as a hundred heels pummel him. He looks for his canine friend, but he can't find him in the throng. "Scooby-Doo, where are you?"

"Rhere Ri am!" Scooby replies. He pops up with an ice cream cone, a corn dog, and a slice of pizza in his paws. "Rummy!"

"Like, where's everybody going? Did a new food stand open?" Shaggy asks, confused.

"Ruh-ruh-ruh roh!" Scooby-Doo stutters. "Rat's rhy! Rook!"

Scooby points with his paw.

Turn to page 22.

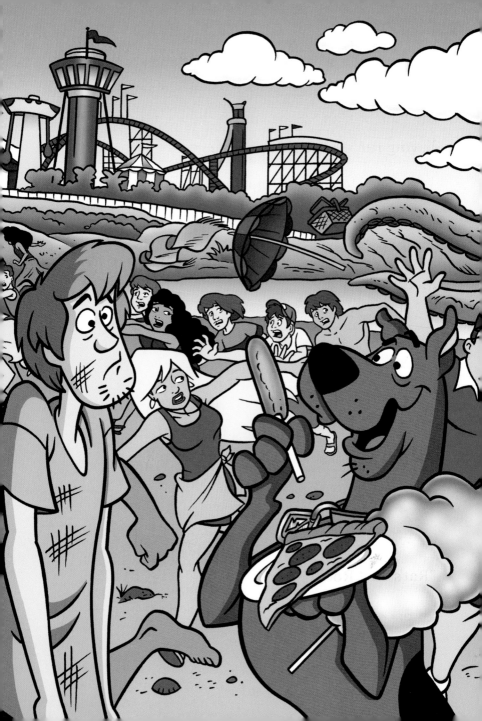

Shaggy stares down the beach and sees what Scooby is pointing at.

A giant eyeball stares down at them, and it belongs to an even bigger sea monster! Thick tentacles grip and crush the vendor stands as the creature crawls along the boardwalk.

There's only one thing Shaggy and Scooby-Doo can do!

"Zoinks!" says Shaggy. "Like, run, Scoobs!"

WHOOSH!

The two friends take off in a flash. They flee so fast that they don't have time to think—what's a sea monster doing on land? The only thing on their minds is escape!

Scooby and Shaggy are so frazzled they don't think straight. They don't follow the rest of the crowd running away from the monster. They run in the opposite direction!

The monster chases them into the nearby amusement park.

"He's after us!" Shaggy yells. "Faster, Scoobs! We need to outrun this crazy creature!"

Scooby-Doo shakes his head like a wet dog. "Ride! Ride!" he suggests instead.

If Shaggy & Scooby find a place to hide, turn to page 68.
If Shaggy & Scooby keep running, turn to page 94.

Daphne lowers her kiteboard to the water below, but she can't escape the sea monster. The kite gets tangled in the sea monster's extra-long tentacles. They whip her around and around until she is dizzy.

To make matters worse, a swarm of police and Coast Guard helicopters buzz the monster. It swats at them with its tentacles, including the ones that have Daphne snared.

"This is going to give me whiplash," Daphne says. "I have to get myself out of this. But how?"

WHOOSH! Another strong gust of wind fills Daphne's kite. The fabric billows. The nylon lines pull at Daphne's harness. The kite pulls the sea monster sideways, too. It isn't very much, but it gives Daphne an idea!

"Those helicopters will come in handy," she says. Daphne waves at them to come closer. "Help! Help! Save me from this monster!"

THWOOP! THWOOP! THWOOP!

A large Coast Guard chopper soars toward Daphne. She can see a rescue diver in the open hatch and feel the buffeting wind caused by the turning rotors. The canopy of Daphne's sail swells, and the monster is dragged along behind it like a kitesurfer.

But Daphne's not safe yet. The monster is heading for a sea cliff!

Turn to page 33.

Fred can't resist the temptation to reach out and touch the sea monster. He is surprised to discover that its skin isn't skin at all. It's plastic! He pinches the monster. It doesn't react.

Well, what do you know? This monster is a machine! Fred concludes. *That's a relief.*

Suddenly, the water churns as the monster starts to swim away from the reef. Fred grabs onto one of the tentacles. He wants to find out who is behind this maritime menace.

Fred worries. *I just hope I can hold my breath long enough to solve this mystery!*

If Fred is carried out to sea, turn to page 27.
If Fred is carried deeper under water, turn to page 40.

The monster carries Fred out to sea. It travels at a tremendous speed. Fred can barely hold on, and he is running out of breath!

If I let go now, I'm doomed! Fred thinks. *I must be in the middle of the ocean. No one will ever find me.*

Suddenly, he sees a brilliant light in the distance. It's a submarine beacon. It guides the mechanical monster toward a massive underwater building. The monster slows down as it approaches.

Don't put on the brakes now! I'm about to turn blue! Fred thinks. His lungs burn from lack of air.

The monster swims into the building. Fred swims to the surface and sees that he is in a large docking bay. There are small submarines and other underwater vessels all around the large chamber.

Turn the page.

None of them have any identifying marks. That makes Fred suspicious. When he sees armed guards patrolling up and down the docks, he knows something serious is happening here.

"Who are these people and what are they doing here?" he wonders. "Are they smugglers? Pirates? Spies?"

Fred swims over to a ladder. He wants to look around and figure out this mystery. He doesn't get far before one of the guards sees him.

"Halt!" the guard shouts.

Fred does just the opposite. He runs!

Turn to page 46.

"I have to escape and tell the authorities that this monster is a fake," Velma says.

She tries to break free from the monster's grasp, but it's as tight as a vice.

"It's too strong," Velma realizes. "But I'll bet my brains are better than its brawn."

Thinking fast, Velma takes off her glasses and points them toward the bright, midday sun. The polished lenses reflect the light right through the mechanical monster's eye sockets.

The beam floods the machine's high-tech control room. The man inside is blinded by the light streaming in.

"Ahhh!" the man yells. He covers his eyes with his hands to block the dazzling glare.

The man inside the monster takes his hands off the controls for a split second.

Turn to page 31.

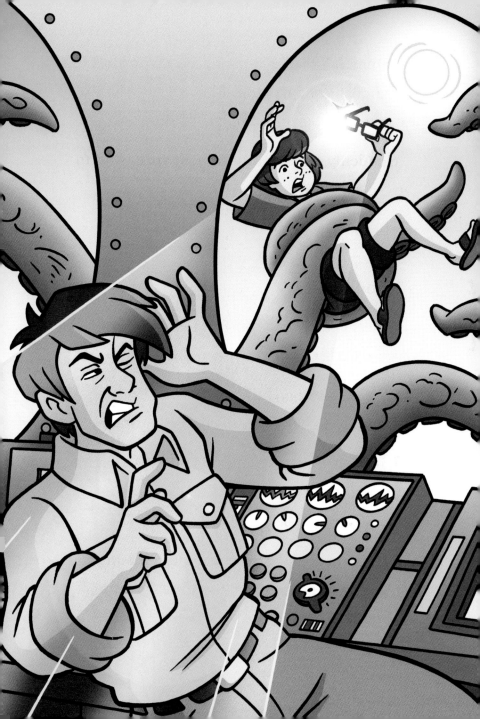

Immediately, the mechanical tentacle releases Velma. Her trick worked! She drops into the water with a big splash. **SPLOOOSH!**

Suddenly, a Coast Guard boat speeds up to her. They've come to rescue her.

"That's not a real sea monster," Velma tells the crewmembers. "That's a machine. A man inside is controlling it."

The Coast Guard officers take Velma to a larger ship. She tells its commander what she told her rescuers: the monster is a fake.

"Fire the nets!" shouts the commander.

The Coast Guard ship fires its net cannon at the fake sea monster.

BOOM! BOOM! Giant nets explode from the ship's cannons and tangle around the monster. Struggling to get free, its head breaks off and floats on the surface, then it starts to sink.

Turn the page.

"Look! There's the man who was controlling the monster!" Velma says. She points at him swimming near the sinking head.

The Coast Guard sends a boat to pull the man out of the water and arrest him. When he is brought back to the ship, he sees Velma.

"You meddling girl!" he shouts. "I built that sea monster to scare kids like you off this beach. It used to be my favorite fishing spot! And I would have succeeded if it weren't for you."

"I hear that a lot," Velma says. She can't wait to tell Scooby and the gang about what she found on her seashell search.

THE END

To follow another path, turn to page 11.

The sea monster is going to smash against the sea cliff! Daphne is still tangled in the tentacles. She can't get out of her harness.

"This is not how I planned to spend my day at the beach," Daphne says.

Suddenly, a hatch opens in the body of the sea monster. A woman looks up at Daphne and scowls at her just before jumping into the water.

"Well, what do you know? The monster is fake. Typical," Daphne says.

The Coast Guard rescue diver drops down on a cable from the helicopter and hangs next to Daphne. He cuts her kite harness and frees her from the doomed monster. Seconds later, it smashes into the cliff and explodes. *KA-BOOM!*

The Coast Guard helicopter lands on the beach and Daphne jumps out. Reporters and TV news crews quickly surround her. They all want to hear how she stopped the sea monster.

Turn the page.

Daphne takes off her kiteboarding helmet and fluffs her hair. She wants to look good for the cameras and onlookers.

"You meddling kid! You ruined my publicity stunt!" the woman from inside the monster yells as nearby police handcuff her. "Those reporters should be talking to me, not you!"

"Hey, Daphne, what did we miss?" Fred asks. He and the rest of the Mystery Inc. gang join her on the beach.

"Oh, nothing new," Daphne says with a shrug. "A fake monster. A daring rescue. Same old thing." She turns to the waiting reporters and winks.

"Yeah, sounds pretty normal," Shaggy agrees. "Hey, Scoobs, let's get something to eat!"

THE END

To follow another path, turn to page 11.

Shaggy drops from the monster's grip and falls into the water.

"Hey, Scooby! Who knew your taste for sushi would save us?" Shaggy says. He looks around for his pal. "Scooby-Doo! Where are you?"

"Rup here," Scooby says from above. He is hanging from the tentacle. "Ri'm ruck!"

The tentacle tries to fling Scooby loose, but he's stuck like glue. All the shaking makes him hang on harder than ever! His eyes rattle in his head, and he starts to see double. All of a sudden Scooby is loose. He soars through the air.

SPLAT! Scooby lands against the monster's eyeball.

"Yuck!" Shaggy cringes when he watches Scooby slide down the eye.

"Hey, rit's plastic," Scooby-Doo says. "And rhere's a guy rinside!"

Turn the page.

Scooby drops into the water near Shaggy. He doggie paddles over to his friend.

"Like, am I glad to see you, pal!" Shaggy says. "You sure had a mouthful of trouble!"

"And rit rasted rerrible!" Scooby agrees.

"That guy and his fake monster are ruining everyone's day at the beach," Shaggy says. "I think it's time we ruined his."

"Ryeah!" Scooby agrees. But then he stops. "Uh, *re?*"

"I have a great idea! Come on!" Shaggy says and swims toward the beach.

"Ruh-roh," Scooby worries, but he follows his friend.

Shaggy and Scooby go to the deserted amusement park. Everyone has run to safety. There is no one to stop the pals from climbing into the park's giant robot mascot.

"Do rou know row to work ris?" Scooby asks.

"Like, how hard can it be?" Shaggy replies. He pushes a few buttons.

The machine staggers toward the beach with Shaggy at the controls. It smashes the lifeguard tower and a few food stands along the way.

WHAM! BANG! SMASH!

"Oops!" Shaggy says. "Like, this is why I let Fred drive the Mystery Machine."

"Rook rout!" Scooby warns. A giant tentacle whips toward the mascot.

"Maybe this wasn't such a good idea," Shaggy admits. The tentacle grabs the mascot. "Zoinks! We're doomed!"

Turn to page 87.

"Help!" Velma decides to shout.

Beachgoers splash out of the water and scramble onto shore, away from the sea monster. No one hears Velma's cries—except the man at the monster's high-tech controls.

"That meddling girl spotted me!" the man shouts. "I can't let her tell anyone."

The man angrily yanks on the controls of the mechanical monster. Immediately, the tentacle holding Velma moves toward the monster's body. A hatch opens! Velma is tossed inside the mechanical monster, and the hatch slams shut.

At first everything is very dark, but soon Velma's eyes adjust, and she can see her surroundings. There are steel beams and sheets of metal on the floor, ceiling, and walls.

"This looks like the inside of the Statue of Liberty," Velma says. "Only this one moves!"

Velma searches frantically for a way out. The hatch is sealed shut. Two other doors—one to her left and one to her right—can be seen inside the mechanical monster.

"Hmm, I wonder where these doors lead?" Velma says. Slowly, she reaches out her hand to grab the left door handle.

Then, Velma stops.

"One or both of these doors could be booby-trapped," Velma decides. "If I invented a mechanical sea monster, I'd set a trap on entrances into my invention."

Velma thinks about what to do next. She decides to take a chance on one of the doors!

If Velma chooses the right door, turn to page 49.
If Velma chooses the left door, turn to page 102.

Fred is carried deeper and deeper under water. He doesn't dare let go. It's too far to the surface. The water is getting dark around him. He's being carried beyond the sunlight zone.

I don't think I can hold my breath much longer! Fred worries. *I'm starting to see spots before my eyes.*

The spots glimmer like stars. Then Fred realizes that he's seeing sparkling metal. The monster is pulling him toward a flying saucer resting on the sea floor!

Sea monsters and aliens?! Fred wonders in amazement. *The lack of oxygen must be affecting my brain . . .*

Turn to page 42.

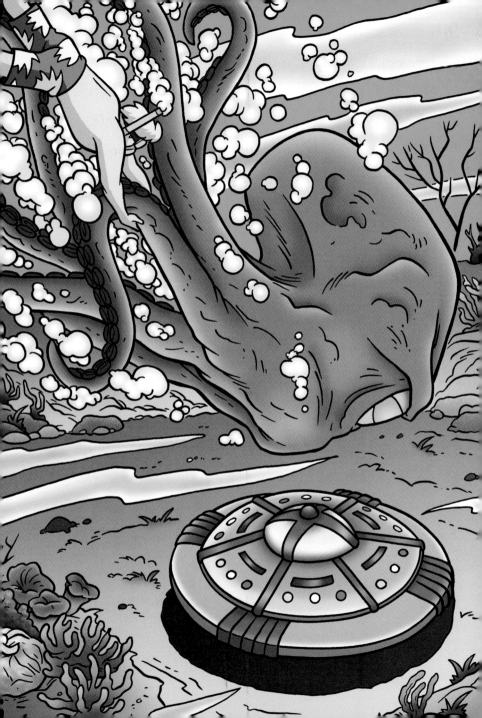

The monster swims through a hatch in the spaceship. There is light and air inside. Fred comes to the surface and gasps for breath. He is in a docking area. Other sea monsters are moored close by.

Then Fred sees the aliens! They are humanoid and have big round heads with multiple eyes. "I hope they come in peace," Fred says. Then he sees they have weapons. "Well, maybe not."

Suddenly one of the aliens removes its head! It turns out to be a human wearing a diving helmet. The eyes are actually window slits.

"The aliens are as fake as the sea monster," Fred concludes. "But what are they up to? Why do they need such an elaborate disguise?"

Fred knows it's time to investigate this mystery.

Turn to page 95.

Shaggy and Scooby decide to let go of the ride. They soar through the air and land on the top of a tall waterslide. The carousel and the sea monster are far below them.

"That was close!" Shaggy says. "We're safe up here, Scoobs. Sea monsters can't climb stairs."

"Ris one can!" Scooby-Doo barks. He points to the monster. It's using its tentacles to climb to the top of the slide.

"That's some sea monster!" Shaggy exclaims. "There's only one thing to do, Scoob."

"What?" Scooby asks.

"Jump!" Shaggy replies, leaping onto the waterslide.

"Scooby Dooby Doo!" Scooby yells and follows his pal.

Shaggy and Scooby-Doo slip down the waterslide to escape the sea monster.

Turn the page.

They barely miss being grabbed by a tentacle.

"Yaaaa!" the pals yell as they plunge down a steep drop. To their surprise, the sea monster follows them!

"It's gaining on us!" Shaggy shouts. The monster speeds toward them like a torpedo.

"Rook out for the roops!" warns Scooby.

Shaggy and Scooby hang on to each other as they go through the waterslide's upside-down loops. They go up, down, and around again. So does the monster. They all land in the giant splash pool at the end of the ride.

Shaggy and Scooby scramble out of the water. But the monster doesn't move!

ZAP! CRACKLE! POP!

Sparks fly out of the sinister sea monster. Its eight tentacles are broken. They are made of metal and wires.

"Like, it's a machine!" Shaggy realizes. "The water shorted out its circuits."

"Rom rea monster," Scooby says.

Suddenly, one of the monster's eyeballs pops open. It's an escape hatch. A man crawls out, and the awaiting police arrest him immediately.

"You meddling kid!" he shouts at Shaggy and Scooby-Doo. "I wanted to scare people away from the park and buy the land to turn it into condos. I would have gotten away with it if it hadn't been for you and your goofy dog!"

"Rey! Who's roofy?" Scooby asks.

"Let's go find something to eat, Scoobs," Shaggy says. "I don't want to tell this story to the gang on an empty stomach."

THE END

To follow another path, turn to page 11.

The guard chases Fred through the strange facility.

Fred ducks through a doorway and quickly shuts the door behind him. He's in inky, pitch-black darkness. Right now that doesn't worry him, though. He's more concerned about hearing if the guard runs past his hiding place.

Fred presses his ear against the door.

"Why is the door soft?" he wonders aloud. **SNIFF! SNIFF!** "What's that smell?"

Fred gropes along the wall until he finds a light switch. When he turns on the lights, he sees wet suits and diving equipment hanging on the back of the door and on every wall. The smell is from damp suits and swim fins.

"These suits smell awful, but they'll come in handy," Fred decides.

"I can use these as a disguise," Fred says.

"Then I can look around this underwater headquarters and find out what's up," he adds.

Fred tries to pull on a pair of the leggings. They are a tight fit, and the damp material grabs his skin. He wiggles and jumps and strains until he gets the pants on at last. He reaches for one of the short-sleeved tops and starts to put it on over his head.

CREAAAKKK!

Suddenly the door opens!

"Who's in here?" a voice demands.

Fred has the wet suit top halfway over his head. He can't see who has opened the door.

"Sam, is that you?" the voice asks.

"Uh, no, it's Fred," Fred replies. "Sam is on a break."

"Uh, okay," the voice says. "Thanks."

Turn the page.

Fred listens to the door close. He quickly pulls the wet suit top over his head and looks around. There is no one in the room with him.

Fred sighs in relief. He goes to the door and peers outside. The hallway is empty.

He is safe—for now.

"That was close!" Fred says.

Turn to page 70.

Velma grabs the door handle on the right.

ZAPPP!

"Jeepers!" Velma exclaims. "That door is electrified!"

It's only a mild shock, but it's enough to stop Velma from touching the other handle.

Velma searches every inch of the metal room, but there are no other exits. No window or trapdoor or air vent.

"It looks like I'm trapped in here," Velma decides. She isn't afraid. "If I know Scooby-Doo and the gang, they'll investigate this monster and find out it's fake. I'll be rescued soon."

Velma sits down on the cold metal floor to wait for the other Mystery Inc. members.

THE END

To follow another path, turn to page II.

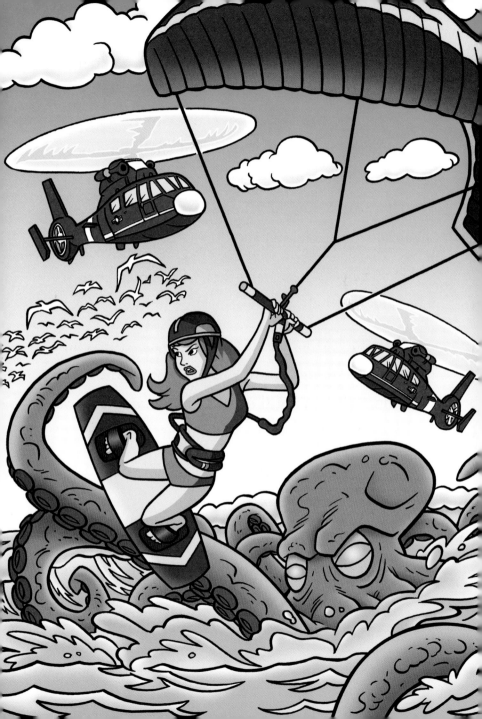

Daphne pulls on the kite's lines as hard as she can, lifting the kiteboard higher in the sky. She banks away from the monster. Daphne is safe from the maritime menace, but she's not out of danger. The wind gust carries her even higher into the air. She flies like a bird!

"Jeepers! I'm not heavy enough to make my kite drop," Daphne realizes. "I guess my diet really worked!"

Daphne worries that a shift in the wind could carry her out to sea or into a sea cliff. She could collide with one of the helicopters flying around the sea monster.

"Or, that flock of seagulls could hit me!" Daphne says to herself.

A cloud of seabirds flies toward Daphne. The sea monster and the noisy helicopters have frightened them. Daphne swerves her kite to avoid them, but she can't get out of the way.

Turn the page.

The birds strike Daphne and her sail. Even though she's wearing a protective vest and helmet, Daphne feels like huge hailstones are hitting her. She and the kiteboard take a beating.

Then she hears a sound that sends a bolt of fear down her spine.

RIIIIP!

"Oh, no! The birds shredded my kite!" Daphne realizes. "I'm going to crash!"

Turn to page 88.

Fred manages to find his way back to the docking bay. It takes him a long time. All the hallways look the same!

"I need a plan of escape," Fred says to himself. He looks around the docks and sees the mechanical sea monster moored nearby. "I know! I'll just leave the same way I arrived."

Fred starts to walk across the dock toward the monster. No one notices him. He is almost at his goal when alarms begin to blare. Everyone on the docks runs—including Fred!

Fred sprints toward the sea monster.

The mechanical monster is not guarded. Fred jumps into the control pod through the open eyeball hatch.

"Made it! Now how does this thing work?" Fred asks himself. "First things first—how do I close the hatch?"

Turn the page.

Fred presses buttons at random. Engines switch on, tentacles thrash, and the eyeball hatch lowers. Suddenly, a powerful concussion pounds the underwater base!

KA-BOOM!

Everyone on the docks falls down. They are all knocked unconscious.

"Um, did I do that?" Fred wonders aloud.

Fred studies the control panel of the sea monster. "Hey, this is as easy as driving the Mystery Machine!" he says. A few minutes later Fred gets the sea monster to the surface.

But he is surrounded by Navy ships.

"Surrender or be captured," a voice is heard over a loudspeaker.

"They don't know I'm one of the good guys!" Fred realizes. "It's time to abandon ship—um, monster!"

Fred leaps from the machine just as it is captured by a gigantic net. He swims away and is plucked out of the water by the Coast Guard.

"Put your hands up!" the officer commands.

Turn to page 78.

Velma is safe behind the large granite rock with her friends. She studies the sea monster threatening the beach. All the people have run away in fear.

Velma isn't afraid. She's curious.

"That's not a sea monster," Velma says. "A creature that shape and size can't live at the surface of the ocean. Not a real one, anyway."

Velma stands up from the shelter of the rock.

"Even a giant squid can't do what that thing is doing," Velma says. "That monster is a fake!"

"Velma's right," Fred says. He shouts to the people on the beach. "Hey, everyone! The monster is a phony!"

"Here, we'll prove it!" Daphne yells.

She throws a rock at the monster. It makes a metallic sound as it bounces off the creature.

Turn to page 58.

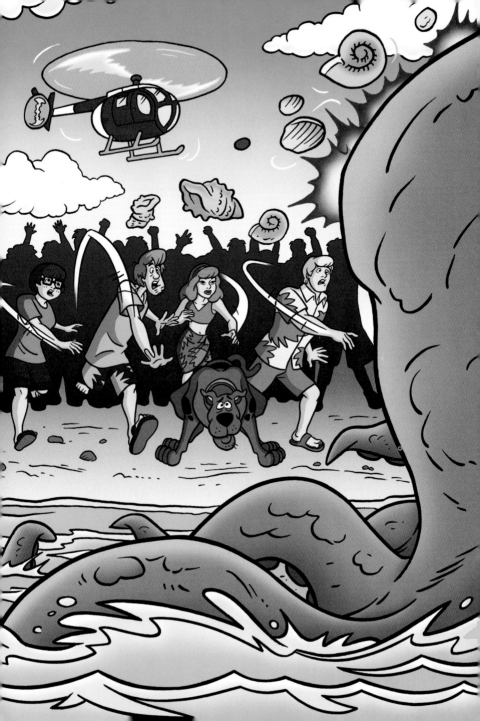

The people on the beach realize that they've been tricked. Everyone picks up a pebble, a seashell, or a piece of litter and throws it at the sea monster!

DING! PING! The objects hit metal.

"Those kids are right!" someone yells. "It's a fake! Get it!"

Moments later, a helicopter lands on the beach between the crowd and the sea monster. A movie director jumps out.

"You meddling kids ruined my monster movie!" he shouts. "I wanted to film real people reacting to a sea monster."

"Like, I think you might want to rewrite the ending," Shaggy says as the police rush in to arrest the man.

THE END

To follow another path, turn to page 11.

Scooby-Doo leaps off the pier and into the water with Shaggy. They make a big splash. Suddenly, there's an even bigger splash. The sea monster has jumped into the water, too!

"Swim!" Shaggy shouts. Scooby doggie paddles as fast as he can. A large wave catches the two pals. "Surf's up!"

The wave carries Shaggy and Scooby toward a sea cave. It's dark and scary, but the sea monster swimming after them is even scarier! They hope they can hide from it inside the cave.

A current drags Shaggy and Scooby-Doo deep into the cavern. They float into a large chamber. There are bright veins of ore in the walls.

"Like, it's a mine!" Shaggy says. "A gold mine!"

The sea monster rises out of the water inside the cave. Shaggy and Scooby climb onto a rock ledge, trying to get away. There is no escape.

Turn the page.

"It's been nice knowing you, Scoobs," Shaggy says, sobbing.

"So rong, ral," Scooby whimpers.

Seconds later, a window pops open in one of the monster's eyeballs and a man leans out. Shaggy and Scooby look at each other in surprise.

"Like, the monster is a machine?" Shaggy exclaims.

"It's a Mining Operations Commercial Krushing Octopod, or M.O.C.K. Ock for short," the man states. "But you two aren't going to live to tell anyone about it!"

The mechanical monster raises its tentacles to smash Scooby-Doo and Shaggy. They hug each other and shiver. This is it! They're doomed.

Turn to page 62.

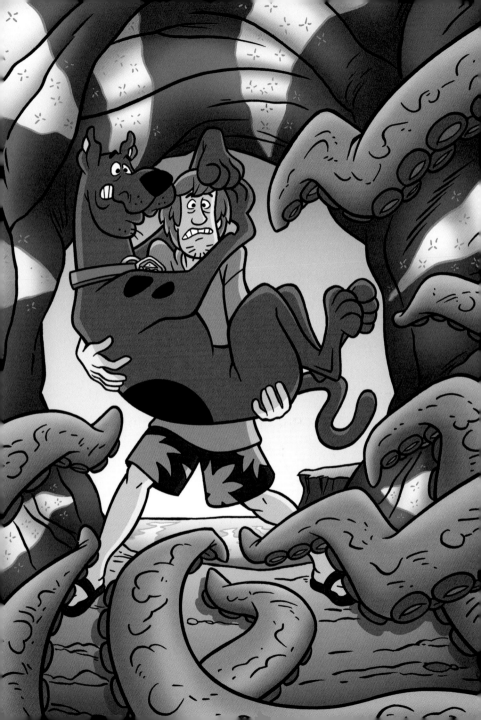

Suddenly, there is a huge crash as the tentacles hit the ceiling of the mine. Rocks start falling on the fake monster. The whole roof collapses! Shaggy and Scooby are safe on the rock ledge. When the dust clears, the monster is buried under a pile of rubble.

Soon, police arrive to investigate the mysterious rockslide. They arrest the owner of the M.O.C.K. Ock.

"My whole operation would have stayed secret except for that meddling kid and his weird dog," the man grumbles.

"The gang is going to love hearing about this adventure!" Shaggy says. "I wonder how many hot dogs this gold will buy?"

THE END

To follow another path, turn to page II.

Velma waits on the beach for help. Other people run away from the sea monster. They stampede like a herd of frightened horses. Velma doesn't run. She isn't afraid. She and her friends have seen stranger creatures.

Velma knows she's in more danger from the frightened people than she is from the sea monster. The crowd tramples right over her. Velma is knocked to the ground. She can't get up.

"Hey! Watch where you're going!" Velma shouts. "Ow! Ow!"

Someone bumps into Velma, and her glasses go flying away. She can't see anything without them! Now she's afraid. Velma must decide what to do—and fast!

If Velma stays put on the sand, turn the page.
If Velma struggles to her feet, turn page 66.

Velma stays put on the sand. She can't see. Waves of people are running by her, nearly trampling her as they pass.

Then suddenly, she hears a familiar voice.

"Velma! You're safe!" Fred says. He grabs her wrist and pulls her to her feet.

"I found your glasses," Daphne says.

"Wow, am I glad to see you guys!" Velma exclaims as she puts on her glasses.

"It's a good thing I wasn't snorkeling when that thing showed up," Fred says. "I might have been monster food!"

"Speaking of food—where are Shaggy and Scooby-Doo?" asks Velma.

"I don't know," Daphne replies, looking around. "We'd better find them."

"I hope they're safe!" Velma says.

The screams of the frightened people running from the beach almost drown out a familiar voice. "Hey, guys! Over here!"

"Shaggy!" Velma shouts. She sees her friend trying to hide behind a big rock and wave at her at the same time.

Fred, Daphne, and Velma sprint toward the boulder. They make it to safety. Shaggy and Scooby-Doo shiver in fear behind the rock. The two pals hug each other as tight as suction cups.

"Scooby! Shaggy! Are you okay?" Daphne asks.

"R-ruh h-huh," Scooby-Doo stutters. "R-rat's a big r-ronster!"

"It might be big, but it's no monster," Velma declares.

"Whaaaat?" her friends say.

Turn to page 56.

Velma struggles to get to her feet. So many people are running over her! If she doesn't move, she'll be squished. Not only that, she'll never find her glasses.

Suddenly, Velma spots her glasses on the sand. And right beside them is the rarest of seashells, the Jewel of the Sea!

Velma studies its rainbow of colors and its delicate, spiral shape. She is so busy admiring the seashell that she doesn't see the huge tentacle coming right at her!

"Watch out!" yells a nearby lifeguard, trying to help her.

THWAP!

It's too late. The tentacle hits Velma and the lifeguard. Velma is knocked to the ground— again! The lifeguard falls on the sand next to her.

Velma gets up.

The lifeguard does not. He's unconscious.

"I guess I'll have to rescue *you*," Velma says. She drags the limp lifeguard toward a large rock.

The only thing on Velma's mind now is escape. The monster's tentacles whip around in the air. One of them slams down near Velma. It barely misses hitting her.

"Jeepers! That was close!" Velma says with a gasp. "Hey, go pick on someone your own size!"

A tentacle smashes the sand on Velma's left side. Another one crashes down on the right. Velma's back is up against the rock.

Right then, something grabs her from behind!

Turn to page 76.

"Ride? That's a great idea, pal!" Shaggy says. He heads for the nearest amusement park ride.

Shaggy and Scooby jump onto a spinning carousel. They try to hide among the animals and benches, but the sea monster isn't fooled.

The slimy sea creature spots them with its giant eye. One of its tentacles reaches for them.

"Rook out!" Scooby warns.

The tentacle grabs one of the carousel animals and uses it to spin the ride faster. The carousel goes around and around, faster and faster. The two pals can barely hang on.

FWOOSH! FWOOSH!

"Like, what do we do, Scoobs?" shouts Shaggy.

If Shaggy & Scooby hang on to the carousel, turn to page 69.
If Shaggy & Scooby let go of the ride, turn to page 43.

Shaggy and Scooby hang on tight. The carousel twirls like a spinning top.

Then, the sea monster stretches a tentacle and stops the ride suddenly. The pals fly off of the carousel, landing on their feet not far from the ride.

"Like, why's the ground moving?" Shaggy asks. He's very dizzy from the carousel.

Scooby-Doo runs around in circles. The canine can't stop himself from spinning. "I rink I'm gonna re rick!" he moans.

A giant tentacle grabs them. Shaggy and Scooby are too confused to escape.

They're doomed!

THE END

To follow another path, turn to page 11.

Fred walks down the hallway. He tries to look like he belongs in the secret underwater stronghold. It works. No one pays any attention to him! Fred peeks into room after room. They are all barracks.

"No clues here," Fred decides. "There must be another level."

Fred finds stairs leading to an upper floor. He creeps up them cautiously. At the top he finds a huge room.

"Jackpot!" Fred says quietly. "This must be the mission planning room."

There are blueprints on the wall. They are designs of the mechanical sea monster. There are also maps of the U.S. coastlines and the locations of Navy bases.

"This is serious!" Fred realizes. "I've seen enough. It's time to get out of here."

Turn to page 53.

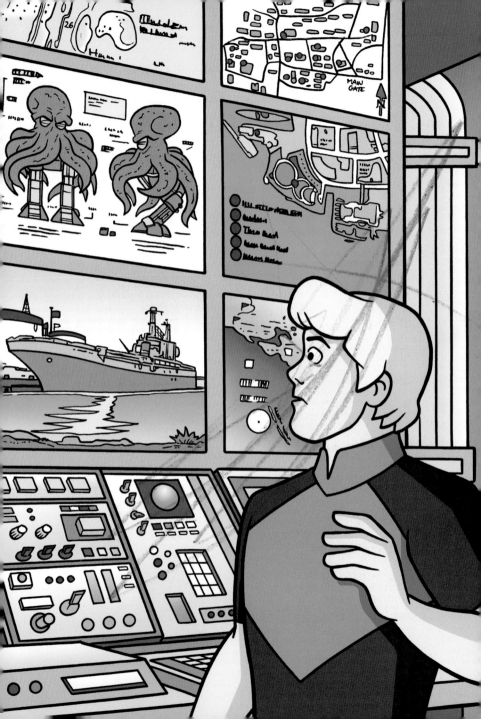

Daphne decides to steer the watercraft toward shore. She grounds the vehicle on the beach and helps Jacks off the passenger saddle.

They watch the sea monster wave its tentacles at the Coast Guard and police helicopters above. The show doesn't last very long. A Navy ship arrives and fires a net at the beast. It's a direct hit! The sea monster is trapped beneath the super-strong net very close to Daphne and Jacks.

"Well, that was impressive," Jacks says. "Almost as impressive as seeing a real, live sea monster."

"Oh, that was a fake," Daphne says. "I see these things all the time."

Jacks looks at Daphne, then at the trapped sea monster, then back at Daphne. He smiles his brilliant Hollywood smile.

"Impressive," he says.

Turn to page 96.

Shaggy and Scooby-Doo drop from the monster's grip. They don't fall far. Another tentacle grabs them. It's the same one holding Daphne, Fred, and Velma.

"Ri, guys!" Scooby says.

"Scooby-Doo, you're brilliant!" Fred exclaims. "You've given me an idea."

"Rho, me? Hee hee hee!" Scooby giggles.

"When Scooby bit that tentacle, it shorted out. The monster is a fake," Fred says. "We have to short out this tentacle."

"It'll open up and let us go, too," Velma realizes. "That's a great plan, Fred."

"Go for it, pal!" Shaggy says.

Scooby-Doo chomps down on the tentacle.

CLANG! ZAP!

There is a bright flash of light and energy.

Turn the page.

Sparks fly everywhere. Instead of letting go of the kids, the tentacle conducts a huge electrical shock from tip to base and back again.

"Yaaa!" they yell. Their hair stands on end.

Suddenly, the mechanical monster stops in its tracks. The shock has blown out all its controls.

"You did it, Scoob!" Shaggy shouts. "You must have hit a nerve!"

The sea monster is not able to stand up. It starts to tip over.

"Ruh-oh," Scooby realizes. "Ris isn't rood."

The monster falls into the water with a tremendous splash! The gang swims away from the wreckage. So does the man controlling the monster.

"You meddling kids destroyed my plan!" he shouts at the gang. Nearby police officers pull him from the water.

"I wanted to scare people away from the park," he continues. "My rival owns it, and I wanted to ruin him. I would have gotten away with it, too, if it hadn't been for you!"

"Maybe the park owner can turn that monster machine into a real ride," Shaggy says. "It was kind of fun!"

THE END

To follow another path, turn to page 11.

Something that doesn't feel human wraps around Velma and pulls her. She fights against it! She holds onto the unconscious lifeguard. The weight of his limp body is like an anchor. Velma doesn't know which is worse—the sea monster's tentacles in front of her or the unknown menace behind her.

"Hey, Velma! It's us!" Shaggy says.

"Ryeah! Rit's us!" Scooby-Doo says. "Re're trying to save rou!"

Velma sees that it's Scooby's paws wrapped around her. He pulls her and the lifeguard behind the big boulder.

"Like, that's a seriously serious sea monster!" Shaggy exclaims. "Where'd it come from?"

Velma barely has time to think about that question. A giant tentacle picks up the rock. There's no place to hide!

"Zoinks! Like, run!" Shaggy shouts.

Scooby's legs spin like a crazy windmill. So do Shaggy's! The pals are so scrambled that they run into each other and fall flat on the sand.

"Whoa! Talk about going nowhere, fast," Shaggy says.

"Ri see stars!" Scooby-Doo says, giggling. "Ris rat the Rig Dipper?"

SMASH! The tentacle throws the boulder to the ground. It misses Velma and her friends by inches. The impact wakes up the lifeguard.

"Earthquake!" he yells.

"Nope. Not even close," Velma says. Another tentacle crashes down. "Let's get out of here!"

The group runs toward the pier. They'll be safe under the timber supports. But the monster comes up out of the water and chases them!

Turn to page 80.

Fred raises his hands in surrender. "I'm not a bad guy," he says. "I'm just wearing one of their wet suits!"

Fred tells the Coast Guard officer about the underwater HQ and the secret planning room he discovered. The officer's expression turns intense. "Take this kid to the brig!" he orders.

"But . . . but!" Fred stutters. He is escorted below decks to a steel cell. Bars clang shut. "I'm doomed."

"I'm a condemned prisoner," Fred moans inside his cell. "If I were Shaggy or Scooby, I'd know what I'd want for my last meal. Everything!"

Later, a Coast Guard officer comes into the brig and unlocks the cell door. "You're free to go," he tells Fred.

As Fred leaves, he sees a group of men in handcuffs.

"Is that the meddling kid who ruined our plans?" one of them shouts. "We would have gotten away with it if it hadn't been for you!"

"They're international spies," the officer tells Fred. "Thanks for telling us their location. You're a hero."

"Wow! I can't wait to tell the gang about this!" Fred says. "Who knew snorkeling could be so exciting?"

THE END

To follow another path, turn to page 11.

Velma risks looking back at the monster. She sees something strange. It has mechanical legs! They have been hidden under water until now.

"The monster is a machine!" Velma shouts. Her friends stop and look. "It might look like a monster on top, but the bottom is man-made."

"That's great to know, Velma—but it's still chasing us!" says Shaggy.

"I have an idea how to stop it," Velma says. She points to a dune buggy parked near the pier.

"Like, this is no time for a joyride, Velma," Shaggy says.

Velma hops into the dune buggy. Her friends are astonished to see her drive straight at the sea monster! She zooms under its legs. The tentacles try to grab her but they get tangled in the legs. The monster ties itself in knots.

Suddenly, it tips over and falls onto the sand!

Turn to page 82.

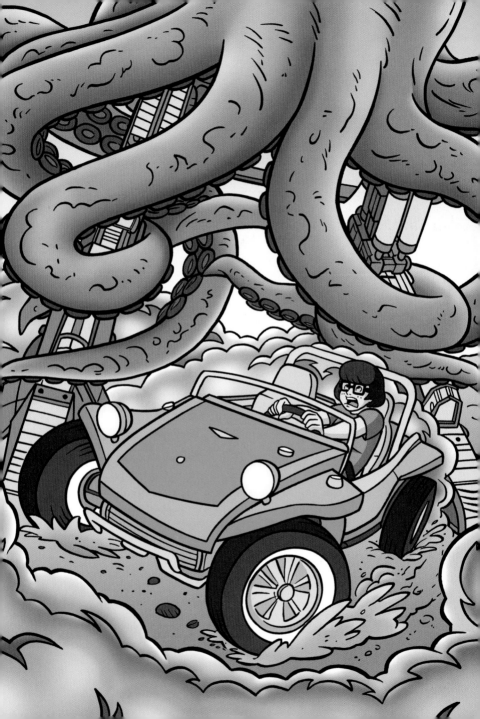

"Help! Help!" someone cries. The sound comes from inside the monster.

The lifeguard runs up to the monster's head. He pulls out one of its eyes.

"Ewww!" Scooby says.

"There's someone inside!" the lifeguard says. "I have to save—her?"

He lifts a beautiful woman out of the mechanical monster.

"Thank you!" she exclaims. "I'm a stunt driver, and this machine went out of control."

"You're safe now," the lifeguard says as he carries her toward the first-aid station.

"Hey, for once the monster was a damsel in distress!" Shaggy says.

THE END

To follow another path, turn to page 11.

Daphne heads farther out to sea.

A giant tentacle smashes down in the water in front of them. It creates a wave that almost tips over the watercraft. Daphne and Jacks hold on for their lives.

"Well, I guess we can't outrun this creepy creature," Jacks decides.

Daphne quickly turns the watercraft in the opposite direction. Another tentacle blocks any chance of escape.

"Aw, come on!" shouts Jacks.

"I'll try to get to those rocks," Daphne suggests. She points to a pile of boulders that are part of a fishing jetty. "We can hide there."

"If we can get there," Jacks says.

VA-ROOM! Daphne presses the accelerator.

"This would be a great action movie, but I don't much like it in real life," Jacks says.

Turn the page.

Daphne steers the watercraft in crazy zigzags to avoid the monster's tentacles.

"We're almost out of danger!" Daphne says, speeding toward the rocks a few yards away.

"Full speed ahead!" Jacks shouts in triumph.

Suddenly, a huge shadow blocks out the sun above their heads. Daphne and Jacks look up and see a giant tentacle descending toward them.

There's no escape from this one!

"Jump!" Daphne yells. She and Jacks leap off the watercraft.

SPA·LOOOSH!

They land in the water with a big splash. The watercraft crashes into the rocks just as the tentacle smashes down on it.

There is a loud explosion!

KA·BOOM!

"That was close!" Jacks exclaims as he floats on the surface. He swims over to Daphne. "Are you all right?"

"I am, but the monster isn't. Look!" Daphne observes. She points to the monster. "It's on fire!"

"I don't know much about sea monsters, but are they usually this flammable?" Jacks asks.

"They are if they're fake," Daphne replies. "It's a machine!"

The flames burn away layers of plastic and foam on the monster, exposing a steel skeleton. Fiery debris lands near Daphne and Jacks.

"Let's get to shore," Jacks suggests. They swim along the jetty to the beach.

Once on dry land, they watch the monster burn, spark, and explode.

Pieces of the mechanical menace fly through the air.

Turn the page.

"This is more exciting than the Fourth of July," Jacks says. A chunk of burning debris lands close by. "Although it might be a tad dangerous."

"Sometimes I think 'Danger' should be my middle name," Daphne remarks. "Daphne 'Danger' Blake."

"Pleased to meet you, Daphne," Jacks replies. "Formal introductions at last."

Turn to page 96.

The mechanical monster tightens its grip on the robot mascot. Shaggy desperately tries to find a way to break free. He hits every button on the control panel. Suddenly, the mascot starts to walk backward. Then it begins to fall! The sea monster can't let go in time. Both machines tip over and crash into the surf!

Shaggy and Scooby climb out of the robot mascot. Velma, Daphne, and Fred run up to them. Nearby, the man in the sea monster crawls out of the wreckage.

"You meddling kid!" he grumbles as the police arrest him. "I was chasing everyone away so I could dig up the pirate treasure under the pier."

"Like, thanks for the tip," Shaggy says with a smile. "Now I can pay for the mascot I just broke!"

THE END

To follow another path, turn to page 11.

Daphne's kite is cut to ribbons, tearing apart in midair. Daphne drops like a stone and hits the water with a splash. The shredded kite floats down from above and settles on top of her. The fabric soaks up the seawater and becomes very heavy. It starts to drag her down!

"I'd better get out from under this kite or I'll end up on the bottom," Daphne says. She tries to swim through one of the rips in the canopy but the kite lines are twisted around her legs. She can barely move. "I'm trapped!"

Daphne begins to sink!

"Hello, miss. Need a hand?" a nearby voice says. Daphne is under the kite canopy and can't see who it is. It doesn't matter to her. She needs help—and fast!

"Yes, please," Daphne replies. "I'm tangled in my kite lines."

"That's an easy fix," the voice declares.

RIIIIP!

This time, the tearing sound is good news. The kite's fabric is cut away, and Daphne is saved from drowning. She looks up at her rescuer and almost chokes.

"You . . . you," Daphne sputters in surprise.

"Take it easy, miss. I've got you," the rescuer says. He reaches down and grabs her wrist to keep her from sinking.

Daphne recognizes him. He's one of the celebrities she wanted to see at the beach!

"Thank you, sir," Daphne says shyly.

The famous actor takes a pocketknife and cuts the kite lines tangled around her legs. "Sir? Please! Call me Jacks. It's short for—" he starts.

"I know," Daphne blurts as he lifts her onto the watercraft. "Hold on, I'm driving."

Turn the page.

"Right then. Formal introductions later," Jacks says, taking his place on the back of the watercraft. "It looks like there's a sea monster menacing the good people of Wild-World Beach. I've been in loads of action films, but I've never seen the likes of this before!"

"I see this sort of thing all the time," Daphne says, sighing.

Jacks doesn't hear her over the roar of the watercraft's engine.

FWOOOOSH!

"Head farther out to sea!" shouts Jacks. "We can outrun this creepy creature."

"Don't you think we should head to shore instead?" says Daphne, punching the accelerator. "We'll be safer on land."

"The choice is yours," says Jacks.

If Daphne heads toward shore, turn to page **72**.
If Daphne heads farther out to sea, turn to page **83**.

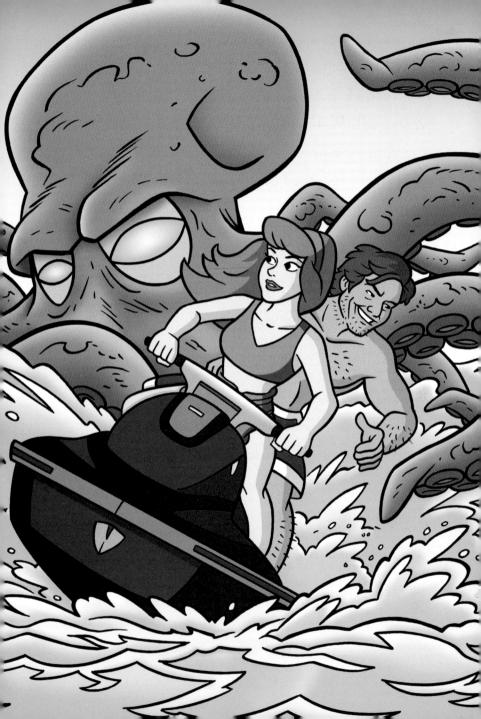

The room is filled with treasure! There are golden plates hanging on the wall and a shoulder-high pile of jewels in a corner. Next to it is a stack of silver-plated armor and a pot of gold coins. Fred is stunned by the sight.

"Wow!" Fred exclaims. "This isn't a spaceship, it's a treasure hunt!"

"Hey, you! What are you doing in here?" a man shouts. It's one of the treasure hunters.

Fred doesn't reply. He runs!

Fred tries to get back to the docking bay. He wants to use one of the sea monster subs to make his escape. Guards block his path. Desperate, Fred locks himself in the maintenance room. It's full of pipes and machinery.

"I need a plan!" Fred says. "I need to distract the guards so I can escape. But how?"

Suddenly, Fred sees the solution. There is a thick steel door labeled Emergency Exit.

"Well, this is an emergency and I need an exit," Fred shrugs. He turns the large metal wheel on the hatch. "I just hope I can get this open!"

SPLOOOOSH!

The door flies open with a tremendous gush of water. Electrical systems blow up and the lights go out! Fred takes a deep breath and swims.

Turn to page 105.

Shaggy and Scooby-Doo run through the amusement park trying to hide from the sea monster. It doesn't give up the chase. Its tentacles whip the air trying to grab them.

"We're doomed!" Shaggy says.

"Ri'm too roung to rie!" Scooby moans.

The pals flee from the monster past the carousel and the waterslide, past the roller coaster and the Ferris wheel. Then they do it again. And again.

Like, weren't we just here? Shaggy wonders.

Suddenly, there is nowhere else to run. They've reached the end of the amusement park.

"Zoinks! We're at the end of the pier," Shaggy says. Waves crash against the dangerous rocks below. "We're trapped!"

"Roh no re're not!" Scooby-Doo declares. He grabs his friend and jumps!

Turn to page 59.

A man climbs out of the sea monster that brought Fred to the ship. He goes through a doorway. Fred decides to follow. He disguises himself in a maintenance jumpsuit and grabs a rusted toolbox.

No one notices Fred as he wanders through the so-called spaceship. He discovers bedrooms, a cafeteria, and a maintenance room, but nothing reveals the purpose of the place. Then Fred comes to a door labeled Treasure Room.

"What kind of treasure?" Fred wonders. He peeks inside. *GASP!*

Fred can barely believe his eyes!

Turn to page 92.

From the beach, Daphne and Jacks watch the sea monster break apart. The creature is made of metal and plastic. Daphne was right about it being a fake.

"This would make a great action movie," Jacks says. "Starring me, of course."

"My life is an action movie!" Daphne laughs. "And if there's one thing I've learned, it's that there are no *real* monsters."

"Daphne! Are you all right?" Velma shouts as she and the rest of the gang run toward her.

"We saw your kiteboard and then that monster!" Fred says.

"Fake monster," Daphne tells her friends.

"Like, not again. Why can't we have a normal day at the beach?" Shaggy says.

"I might have to reconsider the definition of normal," Jacks comments.

A man staggers out of the surf near Jacks and the gang. "My monster. My beautiful monster—ruined!" he cries. Then he sees Scooby and the gang standing nearby. "You meddling kids, it's all your fault!"

"What did we do?" Velma protests.

"Like, we just got here," Shaggy adds.

"You're the one driving a giant machine around and scaring people," Daphne points out.

"This bloke must have knocked his noggin. His reasoning is all out of whack," Jacks says. He waves at a squad of police driving down the beach. They quickly arrest the crazy culprit.

"I wonder why that bloke built that monster?" Jacks says as the police drive away. "Why threaten people? What did he have to gain?"

"Revenge, greed, jealousy, a childhood rivalry," Daphne counts on her fingers.

Turn the page.

"We've seen just about everything, haven't we, gang?" Daphne asks.

"Ryeah!" Scooby agrees.

"You've got a talking dog?!" Jacks exclaims. "Now I've seen everything!"

"Scooby-Doo is one-of-a-kind," Daphne says.

"I could say the same about you," Jacks tells Daphne with a Hollywood smile. "Why don't we have dinner? I know a great seafood place."

"I'd love to!" Daphne replies.

The gang watches Jacks and Daphne walk down the beach arm-in-arm.

"Well, Daphne got her celebrity sighting!" Velma remarks.

"And dinner, too!" Shaggy sighs. "Lucky girl!"

THE END

To follow another path, turn to page 11.

Shaggy and Scooby investigate the screams.

"Wow! It sounds like people are having a lot of fun," Shaggy says. "They sure are yelling!"

"Rook! Rit's a ride!" Scooby shouts. He points to a giant sea monster in the water. There are people in its tentacles screaming their lungs out.

"It must be new. Groovy!" Shaggy says. "Let's check it out!"

The pals run down to the beach to get on the ride. The beach is empty.

"Hey, like, we're in luck, Scoob. There's no line!" Shaggy says with a laugh.

"How do re get on?" Scooby asks.

Suddenly, a large tentacle reaches out and grabs Scooby and Shaggy. They are carried high into the air!

"Cool! Automatic pickup!" Shaggy exclaims. "Like, this is real high-tech."

Turn to page 101.

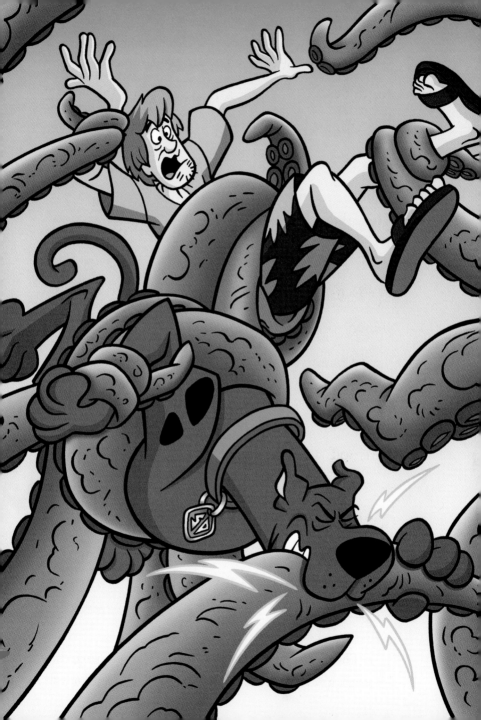

They see Daphne, Fred, and Velma in one of the tentacles, screaming and waving wildly at them. Shaggy waves back. He and Scooby are happy on the ride—until the tentacle starts to squeeze too tight.

"Hey, that hurts. Who's running this ride?" Shaggy gasps.

"Gulp! Ris is a real rea monster!" Scooby says.

Shaggy realizes his friends are screaming in fear, not amusement. He starts screaming, too. Scooby opens his mouth to yell, but the hungry hound has another thought.

"Seafood," he says and chomps on the tentacle.

CLANG! Scooby's teeth hit metal. The monster is mechanical! **ZAP!** Sparks fly from the tentacle. It opens up and releases Shaggy and Scooby.

If Shaggy & Scooby fall to the water, turn to page 35.
If Shaggy & Scooby twist in more tentacles, turn to page 73.

Velma grabs the door handle on the left.

"I can't believe it!" she exclaims. "The door is unlocked! Whoever invented this sea monster forgot basic security."

A metal staircase winds up to another door at the top. Velma sprints up the steps. This time, she doesn't hesitate to open the door.

Velma bursts into the mechanical monster's high-tech control room. The man at the controls is startled to see her.

"I thought I locked that door!" he shouts.

"I don't know anything about your evil scheme, but you're not getting away with it," Velma declares.

"You've got one thing right—you don't know anything," the man replies. "What do you know about designing an extraterrestrial terrain vehicle for the space program?"

"Well, a lot, actually," Velma starts to say.

"Nothing!" the man says, not listening to her answer. "My designs were perfect, and I still got fired from the program."

"Jeepers, I wonder why," Velma replies.

"This prototype was supposed to explore strange new worlds, to walk on alien soil," the man continues.

"Uh, so why is it in the ocean right now?" Velma asks. She doesn't really want an answer, but she wants to keep the man distracted. She needs time to study the control panel.

Suddenly, Velma spots the key to stopping the mad inventor's monster!

Velma realizes that the monster might be big and scary, but the controls to this machine are simple and easy. She'll just need to reach the key located on the main panel.

Turn the page.

"It's just like an ignition key that starts a car—or turns it off!" Velma realizes. The teen leaps for the key and switches it off. The mechanical monster slows to a halt.

"Hey! You can't do that!" the man shouts.

Velma doesn't reply. She grabs the key and runs out of the control room. She goes down the stairs and back to the room with the hatch. The hatch is open!

"Geronimo!" Velma shouts as she jumps out of the metal monster and into the water.

Police boats rush toward the monster.

"Another mystery solved," Velma says. "The gang is going to love this one!"

THE END

To follow another path, turn to page 11.

Fred follows the faint glow of sunlight to the surface. He looks around to see how far from shore he is. All he can see are fake alien guards treading water nearby. "That's him!" one of them shouts, pointing at Fred. "That's the meddling kid who flooded our hideout!"

"We were almost finished uncovering the buried treasure. We would have gotten away if you hadn't interfered!" another crook says angrily.

"Get him!" a guard yells.

The guards and crooks swim toward Fred. Suddenly, a pod of dolphins surfaces and comes between Fred and the hunters.

"Thanks, pals!" Fred says as the dolphins carry him to safety. "When we get to shore I'll introduce you to my friend, Scooby-Doo!"

THE END

To follow another path, turn to page 11.

AUTHOR

Laurie S. Sutton has read comics since she was a kid. She grew up to become an editor for Marvel, DC Comics, Starblaze, and Tekno Comics. She has written Adam Strange for DC, Star Trek: Voyager for Marvel, plus Star Trek: Deep Space Nine and Witch Hunter for Malibu Comics. There are long boxes of comics in her closet where there should be clothing and shoes. Laurie has lived all over the world. She currently resides in Florida.

ILLUSTRATOR

Scott Neely has been a professional illustrator and designer for many years. For the last eight years, he's been an official Scooby-Doo and Cartoon Network artist, working on such licensed properties as Dexter's Laboratory, Johnny Bravo, Courage the Cowardly Dog, Powerpuff Girls, and more. He has also worked on Pokémon, Mickey Mouse Clubhouse, My Friends Tigger & Pooh, Handy Manny, Strawberry Shortcake, Bratz, and many other popular characters. He lives in a suburb of Philadelphia and has a scrappy Yorkshire Terrier, Alfie.

GLOSSARY

beacon (BEE-kuhn)—a light or fire used as a signal or warning

extraterrestrial (ek-struh-tuh-RESS-tree-uhl)—coming from outer space

geyser (GYE-zur)—a hole in the ground through which hot water and steam shoot up in bursts

maritime (MA-ri-tym)—of, relating to, or near the sea

meddling (MED-uhl-ing)—interfering in someone else's business

moored (MOORD)—tied up or anchored, as a ship

parallel (PA-ruh-lel)—lying or moving in the same direction but always the same distance apart

phony (FO-nee)—not genuine or real

reef (REEF)—a strip of rock, sand, or coral close to the surface of the ocean or another body of water

snorkel (SNOR-kuhl)—to swim underwater using a tube for breathing

temptation (temp-TAY-shuhn)—something you want to have or do, although you know it's wrong

unconscious (uhn-KON-shuhss)—not awake or able to see, feel, or think

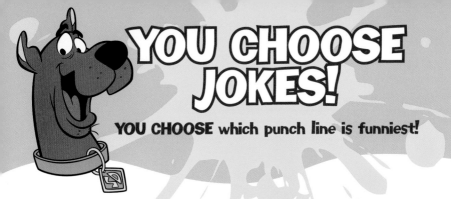

YOU CHOOSE JOKES!

YOU CHOOSE which punch line is funniest!

Why does the sea monster eat lunch by the shore?
a. Because of all the sand which is (sandwiches) on the beach!
b. Because he can't fit in the pool!
c. Because the islands weren't Philippine him up, so he needed Samoa to eat!

What happened when Scooby-Doo accidentally swallowed his flashlight?
a. He barked with de light!
b. Shaggy said, "There he glows!"
c. He was still hungry because it was only a light snack.

Why did the sea monster cross the ocean?
a. To get to the other tide!
b. To sleep in his own seabed.
c. He heard he'd get plenty of mussels on the trip.

Why did the lobster rush out of the bathroom?
a. He won't say why. He just clams up!
b. Because the sardines were filling up the can!
c. Because he wanted to use the paper towels, but he ran out!

What was the ghost wearing when it chased Scooby-Doo?
a. Boo jeans!
b. A boo tie!
c. It was driving a car so it wore a sheet belt!

Why do seagulls fly over the sea?
a. If they flew over the bay they would be called bagels!
b. If they flew over a football field they'd be field gulls!
c. If they flew over the North Pole they'd be icicles (icy gulls)!

What does Scooby-Doo wear during the summer?
a. He wears his coat and pants!
b. Rightweight crows!
c. Nothing, he likes hot dogs!

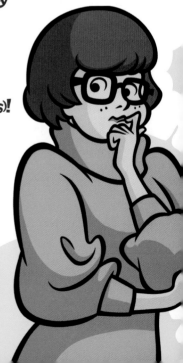

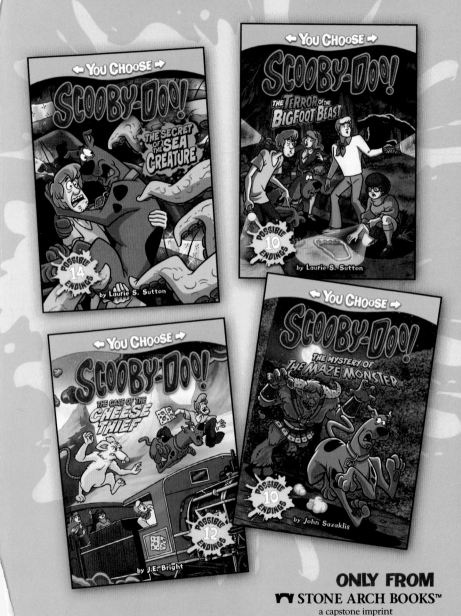

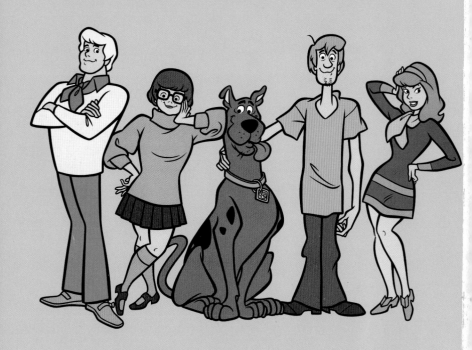